# Inside Yoga

## The Gift of Practice

Lloyd Goldstein

ISBN Number: 978-0-615-38493-1
Library of Congress Control Number: 2010931912
Printed in the USA

Second printing 2024

All Text and Illustrations by Lloyd Goldstein
www.lloydgoldstein.com
lloydgoldstein@gmail.com

Page Layout and Design by Teresa Trubilla
Beyond The Desktop, Tampa FL Trubilla@mac.com

Digital Photography of Artwork by Sam Johnston
www.samjohnston.com
sam@studio4design.net

Print production - William Hoard
BookCreate.com

*Acknowledgements*

Most special thanks to my beloved wife Mary Grace Bronson who has always believed in me, and in the value of months and months of lying on the floor between yoga poses writing and drawing from morning till night. Thank you Mary Grace. I am forever grateful to you.

Infinite thanks to my family, my Mother, Joan Goldstein, Father, Everett Goldstein, Brother, Andrew Goldstein, and Sister, Lori Little for loving and believing in me all these years.

Special thanks to all my teachers, whether in yoga or music, that saw enough in me to help me move forward even when no one was entirely sure if I would ever make it. My Double Bass teachers: Dr. Lucas Drew, Dr. Vincent Kantorski, Mik Groninger, Maestro Francois Rabbath. All my 'family' and colleagues at The Summer Bass Workshop with George and Martha Vance. My friends at The Unitarian Universalist Church of Tampa, my first real audience, who watched me stand on my head, recite, and play the double bass - all at the same time…

…My First Yoga Teacher, Maggie McClain and all the faculty at the Teacher Training Program at Treehouse Yoga in Tampa, Florida. The faculty at The Music for Healing and Transition Program, especially nurse and researcher, Margo Drohan. She knows why. Extra special thanks and praise for my colleagues at The Arts In Medicine Program at The Moffitt Cancer Center: Cheryl Belanger, Carol Shore, Derry MacDonald, Hollie Adkins, Judy Ranney and Kay Plumb for their support and guidance when I have needed it most. Most especially Cheryl Belanger. She knows why. And to Nancy Angard at University Community Hospital…

## *A c k n o w l e d g e m e n t s*

...To all the amazing and varied people who have touched, and continue to touch and bless my life in countless ways each day, and to God for the outstanding privilege of being alive. Thanks especially to my patients at the Moffitt Cancer Center where I am a Certified Music Practitioner playing therapeutic music at the bedside. You are my most wonderful teachers and friends.

Extra special thanks to Teresa Trubilla for sharing her time and skills to create these beautiful page layouts at a time when it would have been very difficult to pay her anything close to what she is worth...

...And to William Hoard for his expertise in the world of color and printing, for believing in the value of my work, and always going the extra mile to make this book beautiful and affordable...

...And to Guerleen Grewal for reading and editing, and Beth Isacke for her ongoing efforts to find just the right publisher.

If I have not mentioned you, please know that you are loved and appreciated, and that we will meet again, perhaps in a meditation, some where and when to be discovered.

Thank you all,
Most Sincerely Yours,
Lloyd J. Goldstein

# Table of Contents

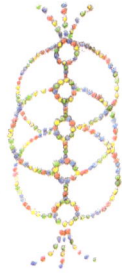

This book contains a collection of small gifts from my emerging consciousness to me. They were born effortlessly into moments of clear space during my Yoga practice.

During the first year of practice 700 pieces of writing offered themselves, almost fully baked, into my awareness. I recorded them faithfully and honestly, recognizing them for the gifts that they were.

In the second year 400 drawings were offered in the same spirit. I accepted by sketching as quickly and innocently as possible. There was little struggle and much joy in this process. I felt rich in gifts.

It is my belief that these presents retain a glimmer of the essential energy/awareness of the moment out of which they emerged: A glimpse of the precious present or the essential "now", the recognition of which, allows us to be most alive and free.

It is my joy and pleasure to share these glimmerings, these glowing embers rising on a column of free-flowing air. May they resonate with some true tone inside you and may you find your own way into the beauty, aliveness and infinite possibilities inherent in your own conscious awareness of the present moment.

Namaste

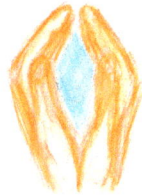

# First Wave

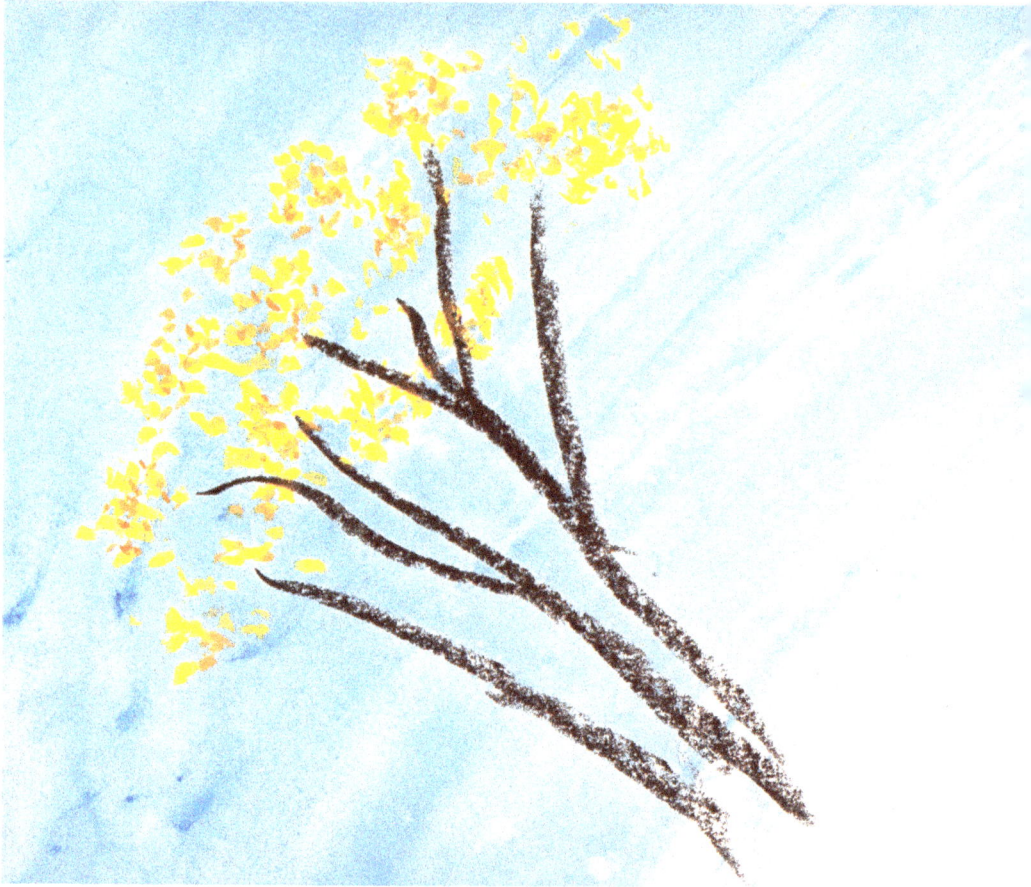

*What is it worth to experience a feeling of rightness in all things?*

*To know that things are moving exactly as they should be,*

*no feeling of haste or desperation, nor lack of anything;*

*To experience each day, each moment, each pose as being*

*born out of nothing, created anew.*

*Today, this moment, is infinitely flexible, possible,*

*pure, potent.*

*It is not what, but how.*

*Not what I do, but how deeply I live.*

*To "live in the moment." What does this mean?*


*To be soft, fresh, open, free.*

*To allow the air to breathe through me, the light to fill me.*

*Colors caress me, energy flows through me.*


*Forgive the worthless past.*

*Slough off its fetid, crusted, useless skin.*

*Feel alive, reborn, capable of anything.*


*Choosing freely, smiling sincerely,*

*Even cleaning the bathroom with ease and good humor.*

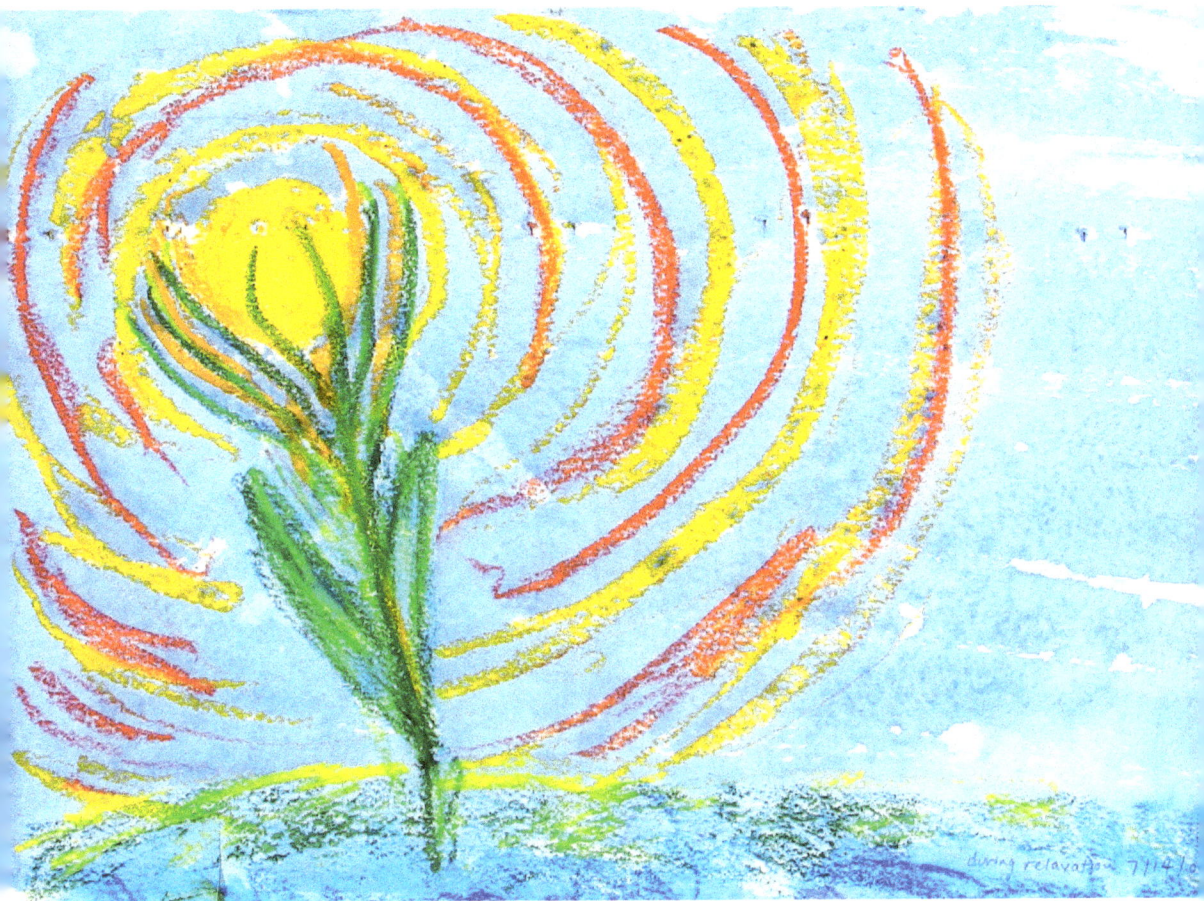

during relaxation 7/14/

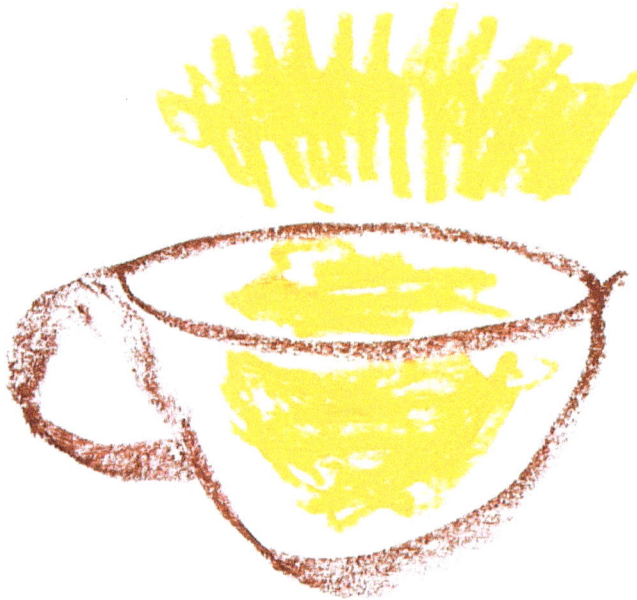

When I look over my shoulder,

stretching my eye muscles to the lower left extreme,

I see my death, clearly and surely.

It will come and I am not afraid, because today I am alive.

I am living the fullness today, so I am not afraid.

I will have missed nothing.

*I enter the temple, sweep out the cobwebs,*

*rearrange the candlesticks and urns.*

*Light shines through colored windows illuminating*

*fine dust motes. It is the beginning*

*of a new day.*

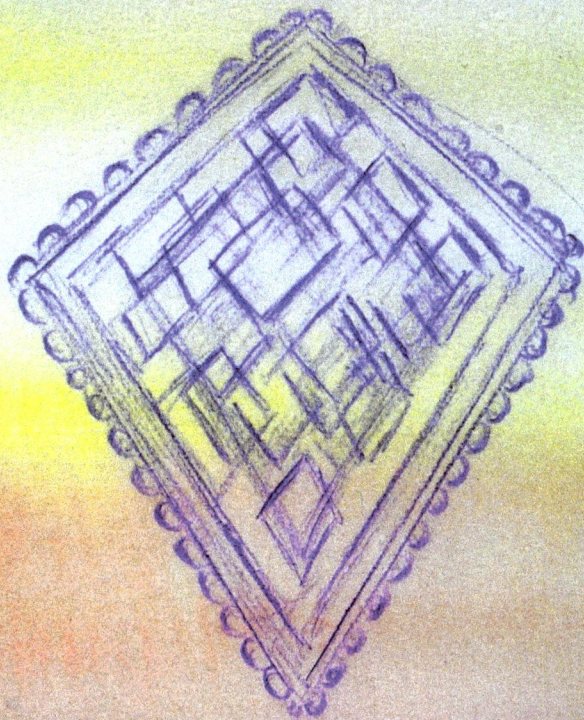

1st light
window on the morning
12/3/99

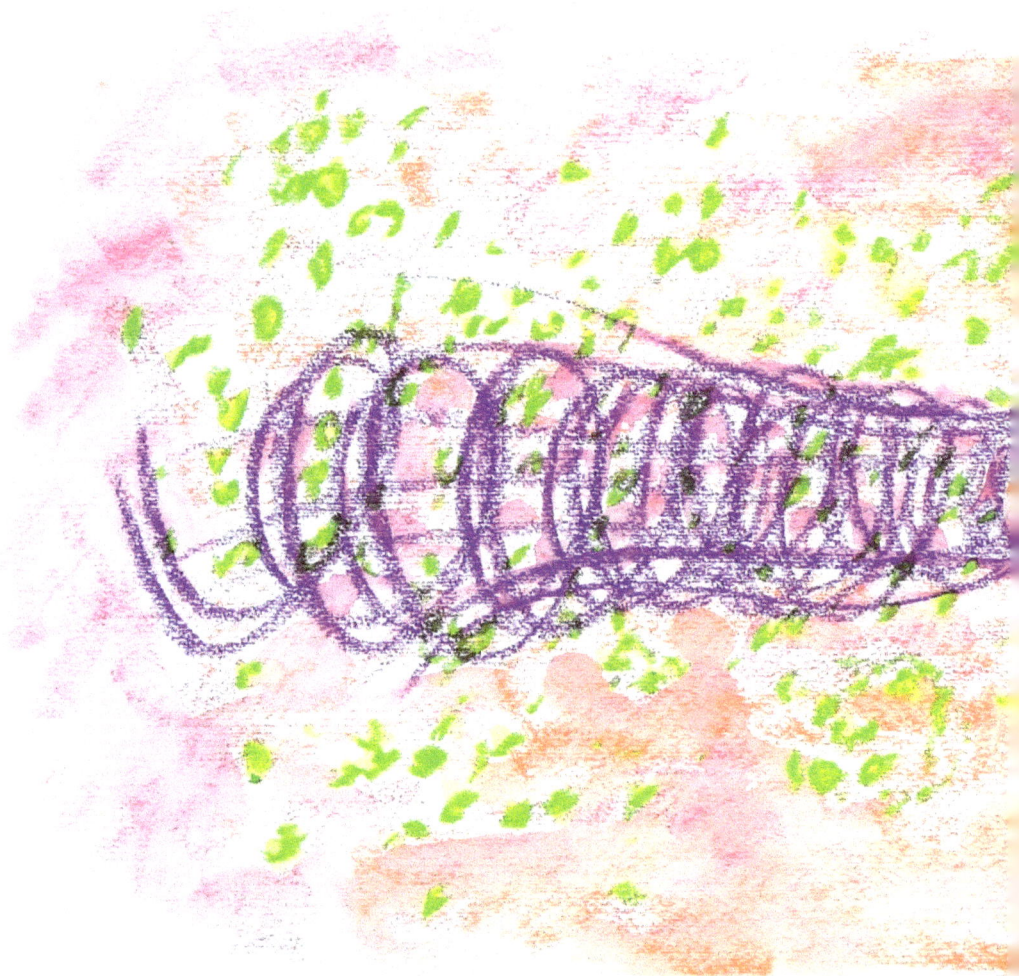

*Firm yet spongy, wafted by gentle breezes.*

*Covered and caressed by bough shadows and*

*leaf-like dancing water diamonds.*

*Bones vibrate, muscles zinging with the earth,*

*turning, swaying, dancing. All this, but*

*having barely rolled my eyes and stretched my neck.*

After Cobra 9/13/00

*Awareness comes like light into darkness.*

*What was dim is infused with light.*

*Where shouted a din there is harmony.*

*Where there was silence is birdsong,*

*squirrel scratchings and softly breezing.*

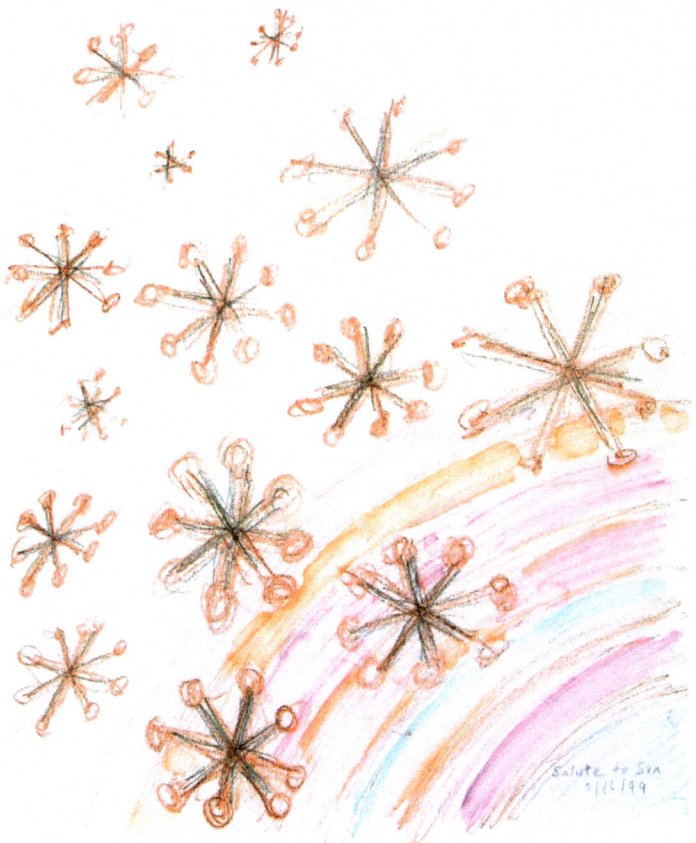

Salute to Sun
9/18/99

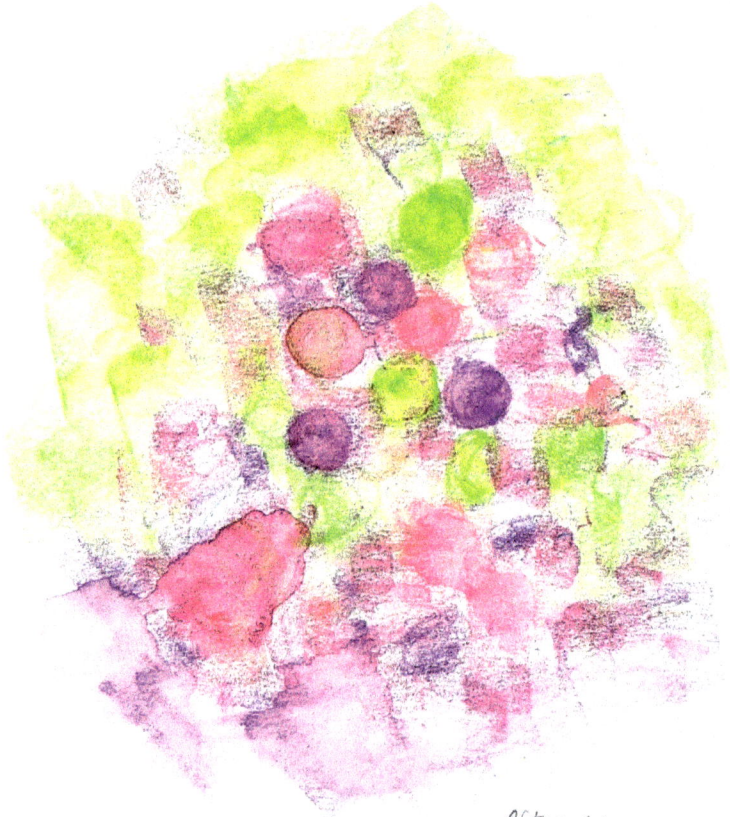

After Cobra

*Why am I always surprised by the light when it comes?*

*Like a grassy space coming aglow as a cloud moves aside,*

*transformation comes quietly.*

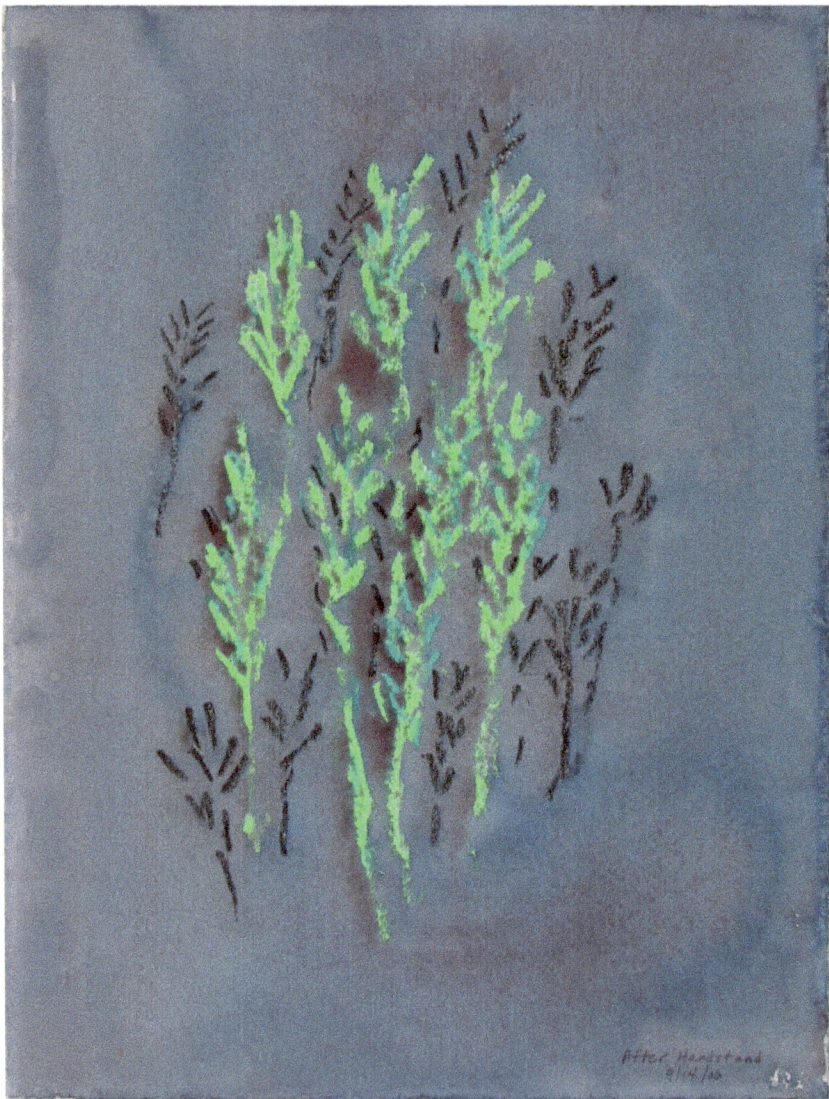

After Hampstead
9/14/00

*After Shoulderstand Cycle,*

*I am a starfish lying on the ocean floor,*

*symmetrical, light, yet firm, and alive,*

*undulating with each susurration of current.*

*In Child's Pose after Headstand*

*I am a smooth round stone basking in the sunlight,*

*leaving my impression in the sand.*

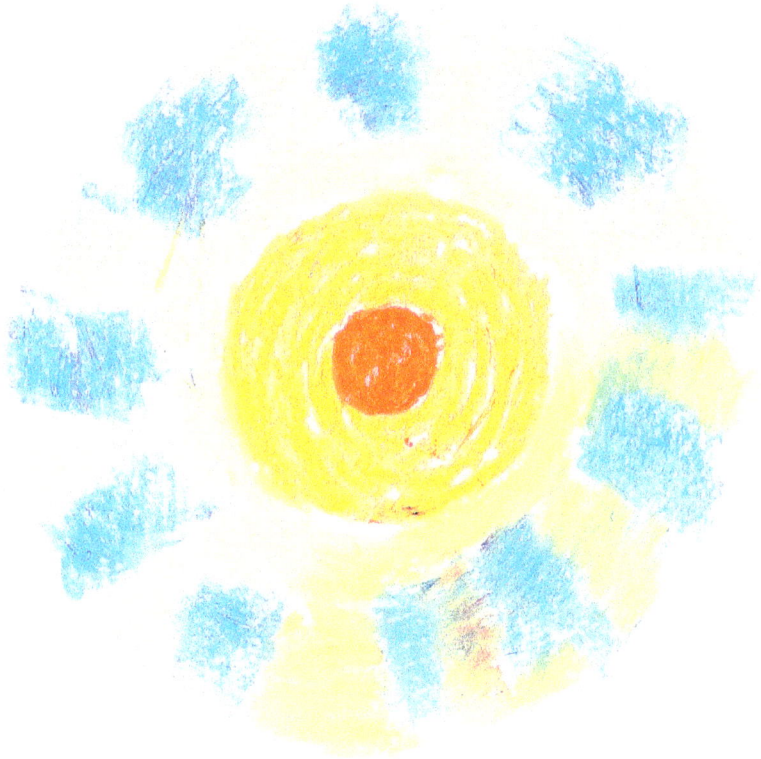

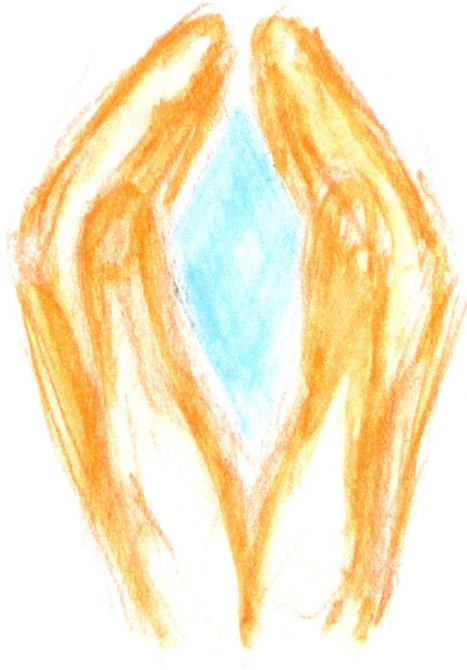

After twisting
10/1/99

*After Bow as I lay resting*

*a blue fire diamond is radiating*

*upward, with an inner fire,*

*upward, upward*

*a blue fire diamond*

*in my chest.*

*What was slow,*
*moves more quickly,*

*what seemed dark,*
*is full of light.*

*That which seemed doubtful,*
*is no longer a consideration.*

*There is spring in my step and a lifting*
*from toe to top of head.*

*I smell the clean fresh air*
*through the cracked window,*

*see the bougainvillea all in bloom.*
*What could possibly be the matter?*

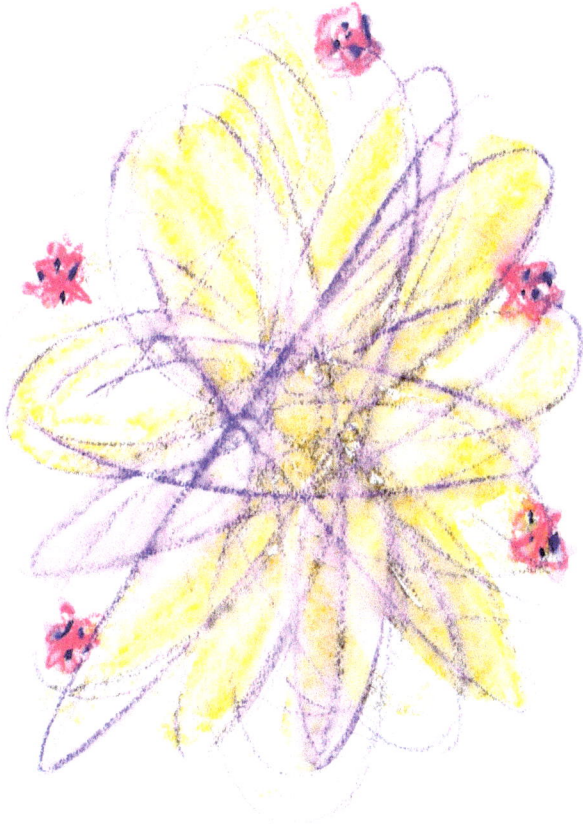

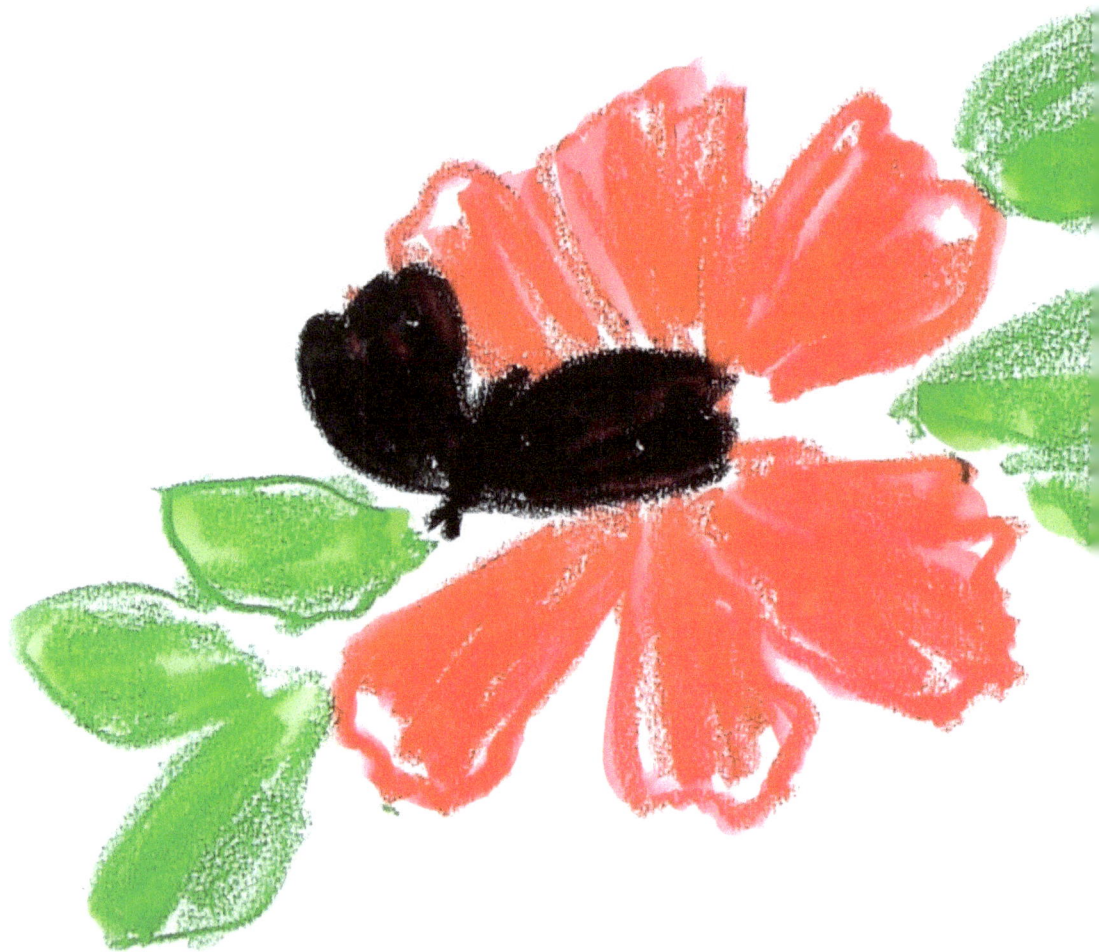

*In Tree Pose today, shoulders move back and down,*

*Chest opens and lifts from below the navel,*

*Arches are strong with weight supported just in front of the heel.*


*And look! I am surprised by the first red hibiscus flower of the season.*


*In is out,*

*Out is in,*

*All is one.*

*In is out and out is in. It is all one. We are all one.*

*Roots reach deep into the earth, where I have been before.*

*Branches reach to the sky where I am, and have been before.*

*There, I go twisting in light and shadow,*

*a strong, muscular oak hosting Spanish moss and squirrels,*

*breathing lightly, in the morning light.*

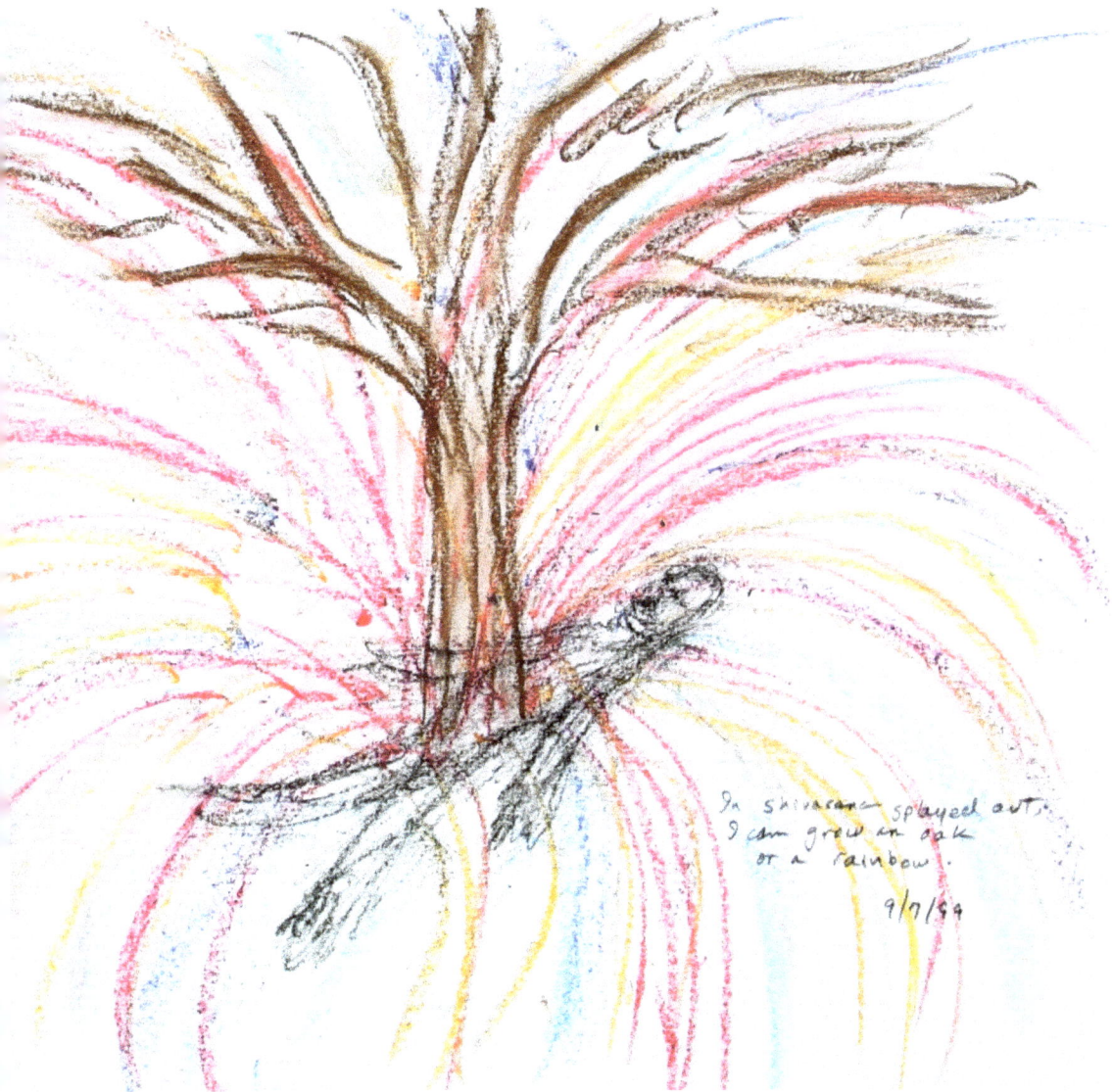

In shimmer splayed out,
I can grow an oak
or a rainbow.

9/7/94

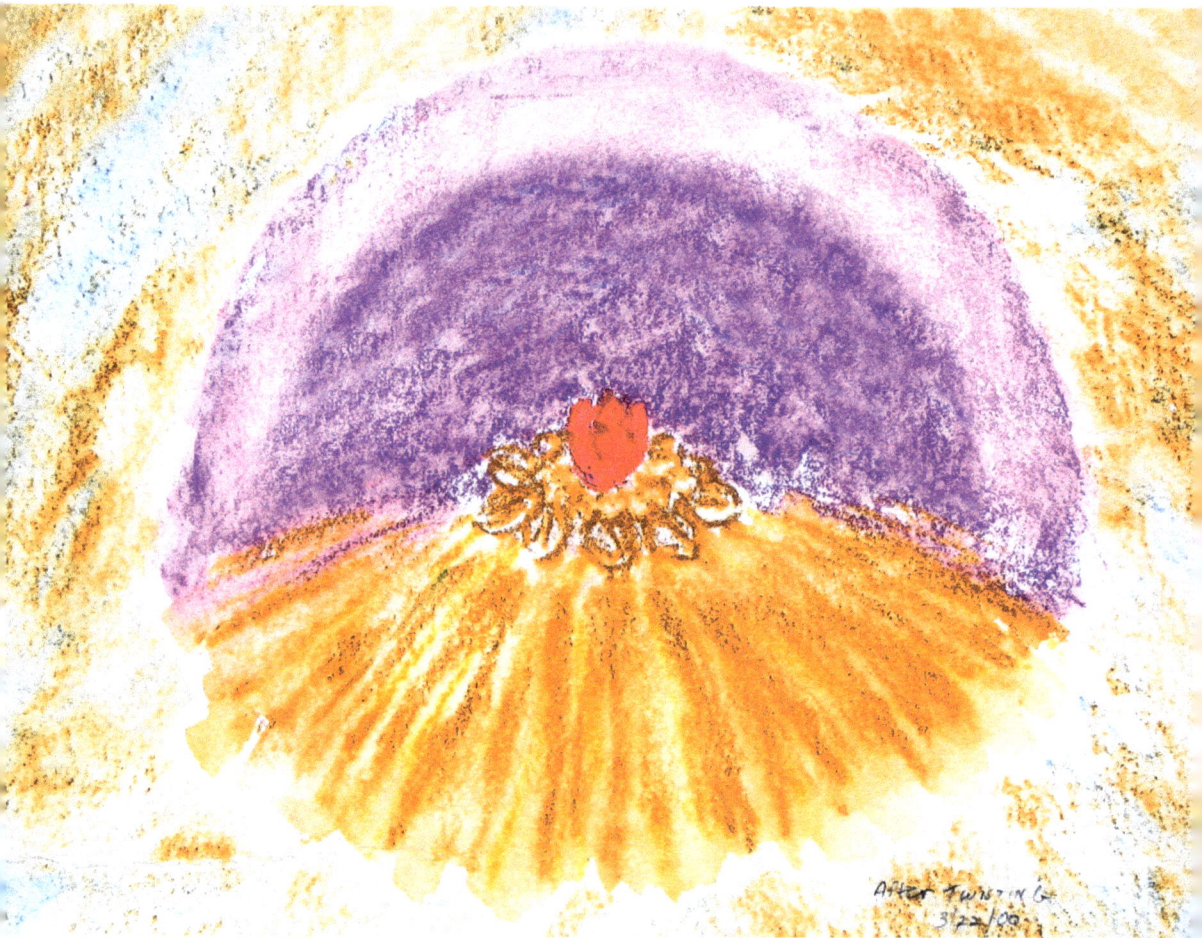

*Each breath, each unhurried movement, brings me back to me*

*and I am rich, when only minutes ago I felt impoverished.*

*Yoga poses, though wonderful for developing physical strength and flexibility,*
*remind us that we are more than our physical bodies, or that*
*our bodies are everything, and much more than we thought.*

*Connections between the heavier, food sheath-body,*
*and the lighter, subtler bodies, are opened*
*and breath flows through spirit and mind*
*in remembrance and renewal of our birthright*
*as free and spiritual beings.*

*Ears unclog and eyes are opened*
*to colors and light that seem brand new.*
*Ordinary sounds of*
*clocks, traffic, fountains, birds and insects*
*become obvious symphonies of subtle composition, the*
*strength of the oak is felt and known.*

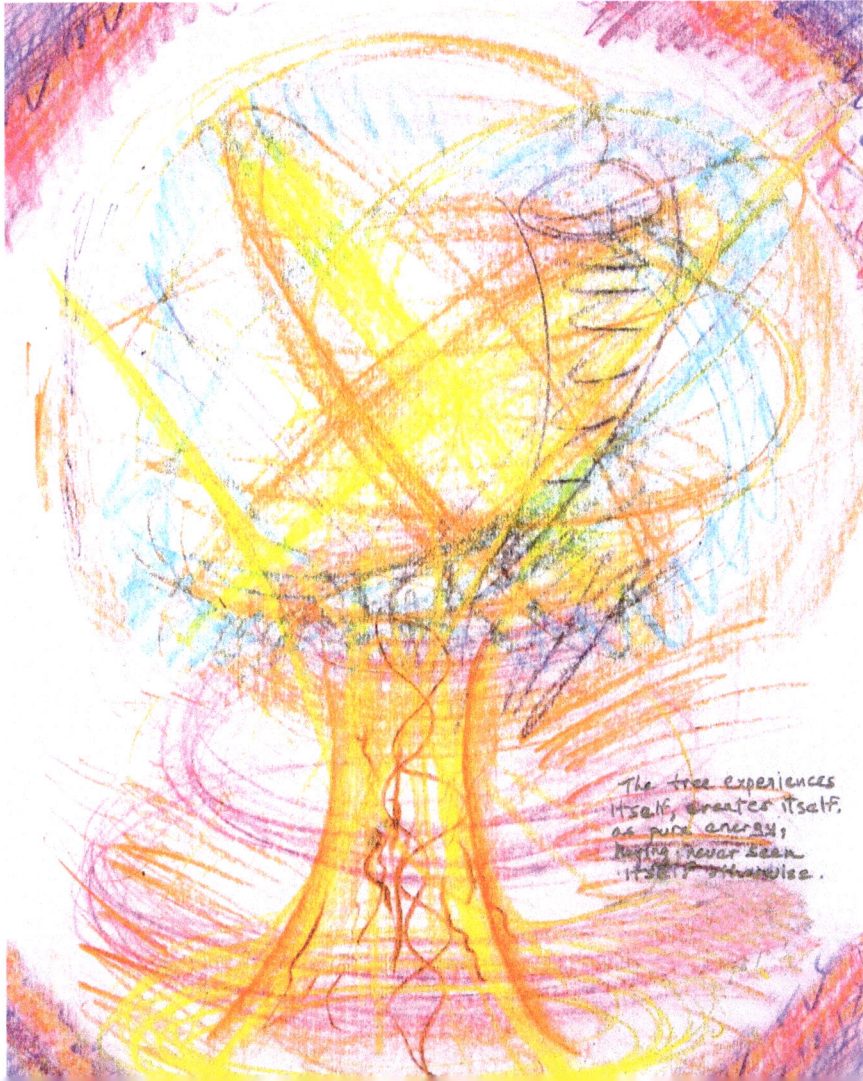

The tree experiences
itself, creates itself,
as pure energy,
having never seen
itself otherwise.

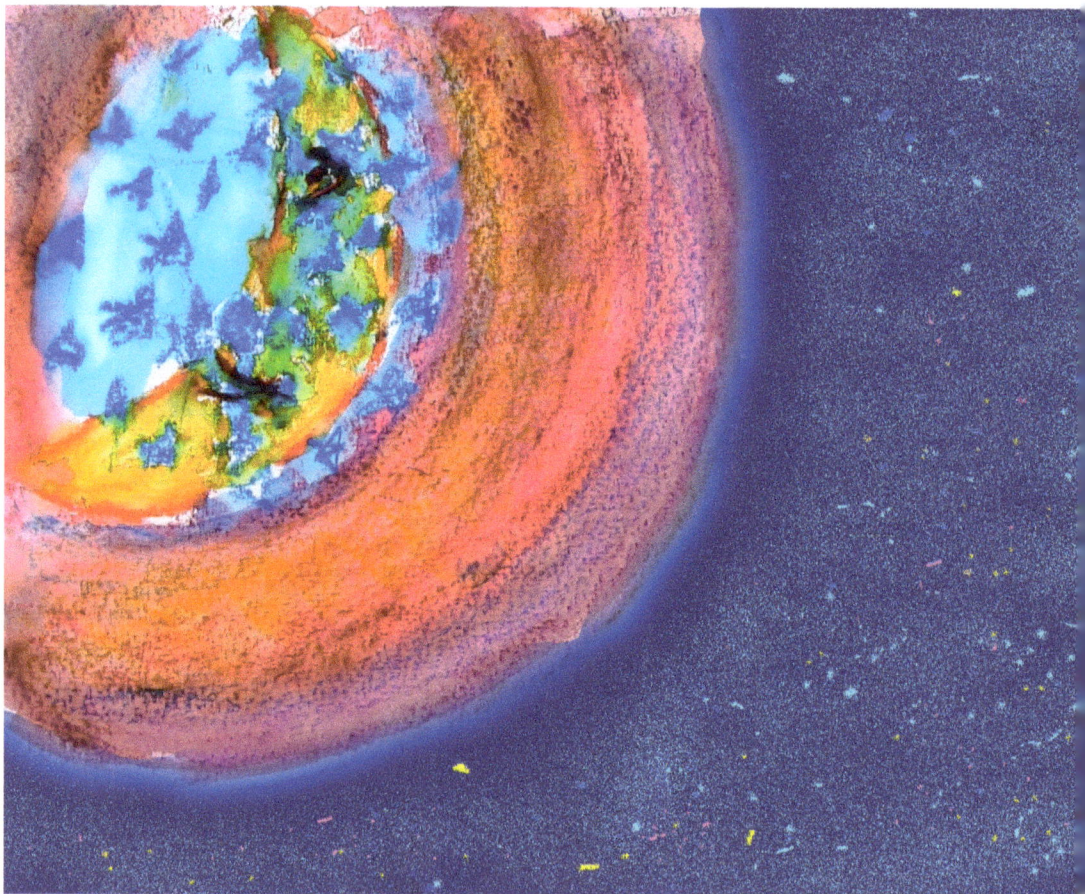

*In Bow, today, my shoulders and upper back are wide and open.*

*I am a bowl, a vessel, a single sacred curve, filling and emptying.*

*Each moment is a joy and a treasure. The smoke of incense*

*wafts gently by, here and then gone, burning cheerfully away.*

*Sitting tall and light*

*i am rising like a young tree*

*feeling again the greenness in my hair*

*and the power in my heart and limbs.*

*Standing, my chest lifts tilting at treetops.*

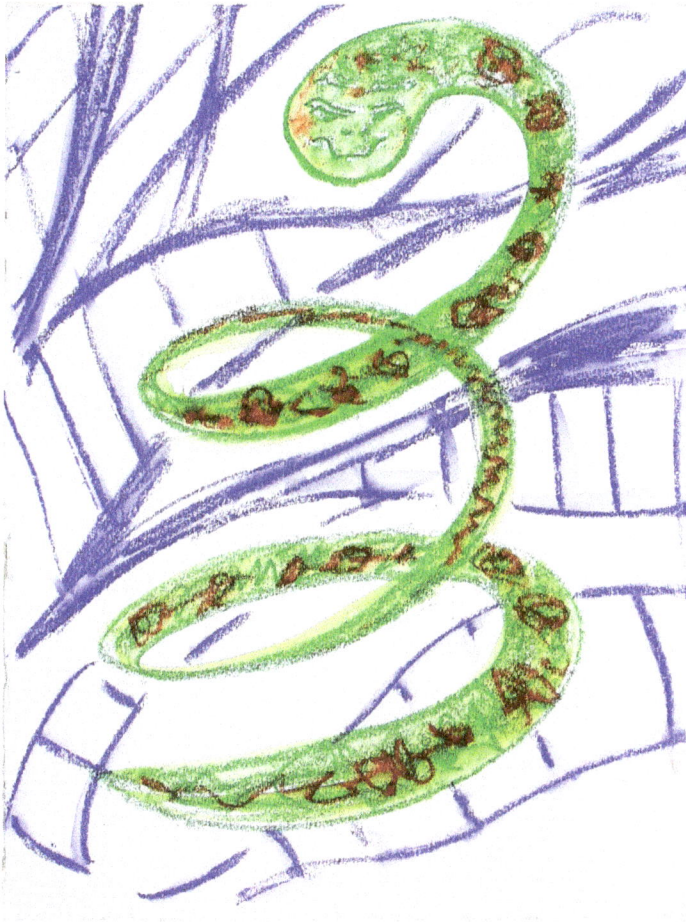

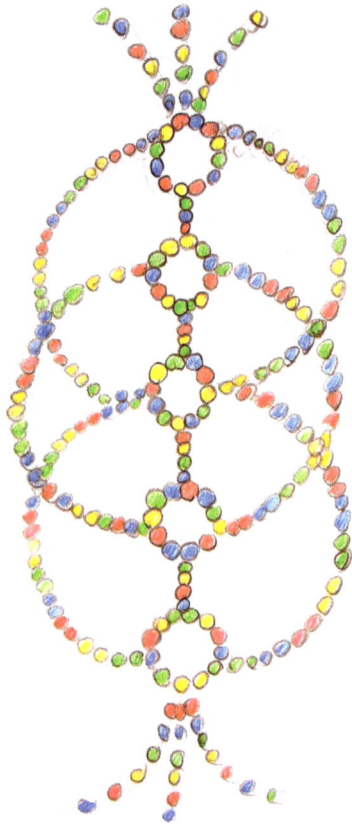

*Headstand is new now.*

*Arms, shoulders and chest lifting into the floor,*

*neck reaching down and through. Afterwards,*

*in Child's Pose, I notice my body smiling inside.*

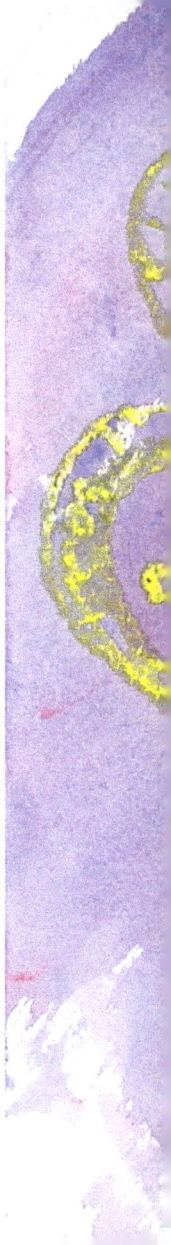

*Death tells me to take time,*

*to be soft, and to*

*listen to everything.*

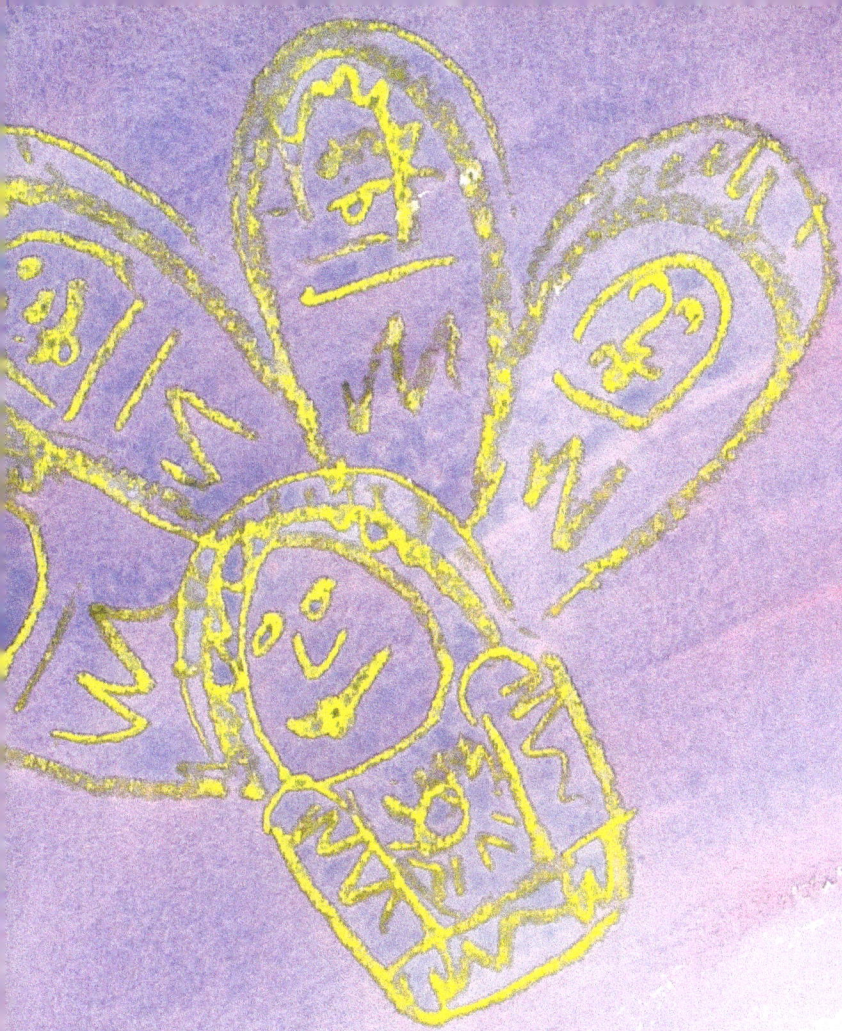

Head and neck stretches
2/8/00
"laughing indian man
headress."

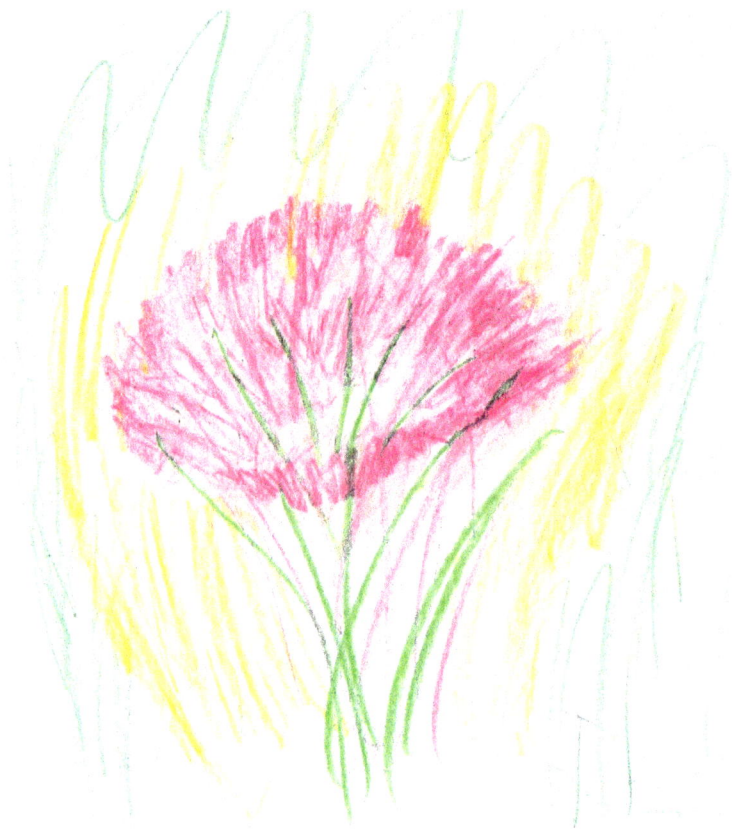

*Inside Yoga*

The main thing is to listen:

to listen with my whole body, my being, my heart.
I listen to my surroundings, and to my heart.

I listen for the richness, the grandeur,
the greatness and smallness,
the solid and the ephemeral.

I listen and I am fulfilled.

*I am grateful to be able to sit tall and be still.*

*In my interstices I am burning,*

*Losing that which I no longer need.*


*A cleansing, golden fire that does not hurt,*

*But glows brightly from within, like a lantern*

*Shining through an intricately woven shell.*


*Garbage is burning away, floating upward,*

*Leaving the lamp cleaner, clearer and brighter.*

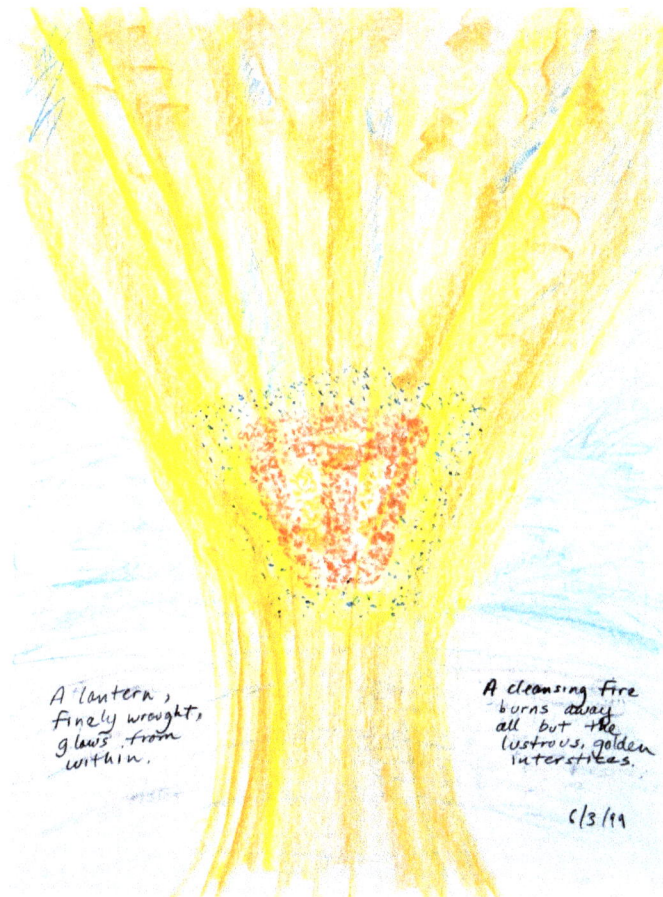

A lantern,
finely wrought,
glows from
within.

A cleansing fire
burns away
all but the
lustrous, golden
interstices.

6/3/99

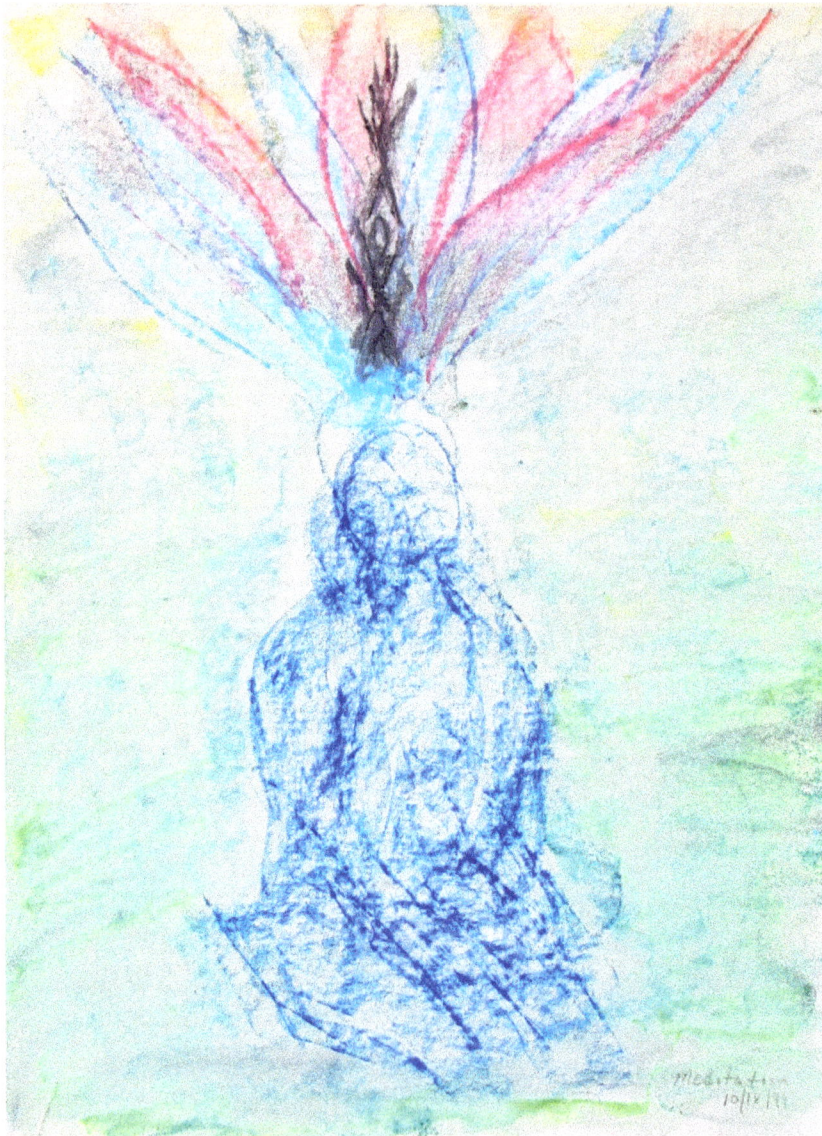

Meditation
10/IX/9?

# Inside Yoga

*I am sitting. Time is gently moving.*
*Legs crossed, back straight, yet supple, wafting upward.*

*Gazing forward, relaxed,*
*outward — inward — balanced.*

*I am devoted to me finding me,*
*to life living itself in my awareness.*

*In these moments strife and struggle are unmasked,*
*their closeness and dimness banished.*

*Whisked away.       d i s a p p e a r e d*

*All struggling and strife are a sham, grasping and greed —*
*distraction from the reality of who I am.*

*I am everything.*

*Fountain filling from bottom to top,*
*A conduit from tail to crown,*
*Open and flowing with energy raining*
*down and up through body's center.*
*Continuously flowing, resting*
*gently in the heart place.*
*Past the automatic breather-heart-pump,*
*past the very important decision maker,*
*to the Joy Body, to the*
*Nothing nowhere everywhere place,*
*where breathing almost disappears.*
*To stillness, to peace and finally,*
*to Love. Gratitude and love pouring, flowing,*
*Radiating outward to people and everywhere.*
*It is infinite.*

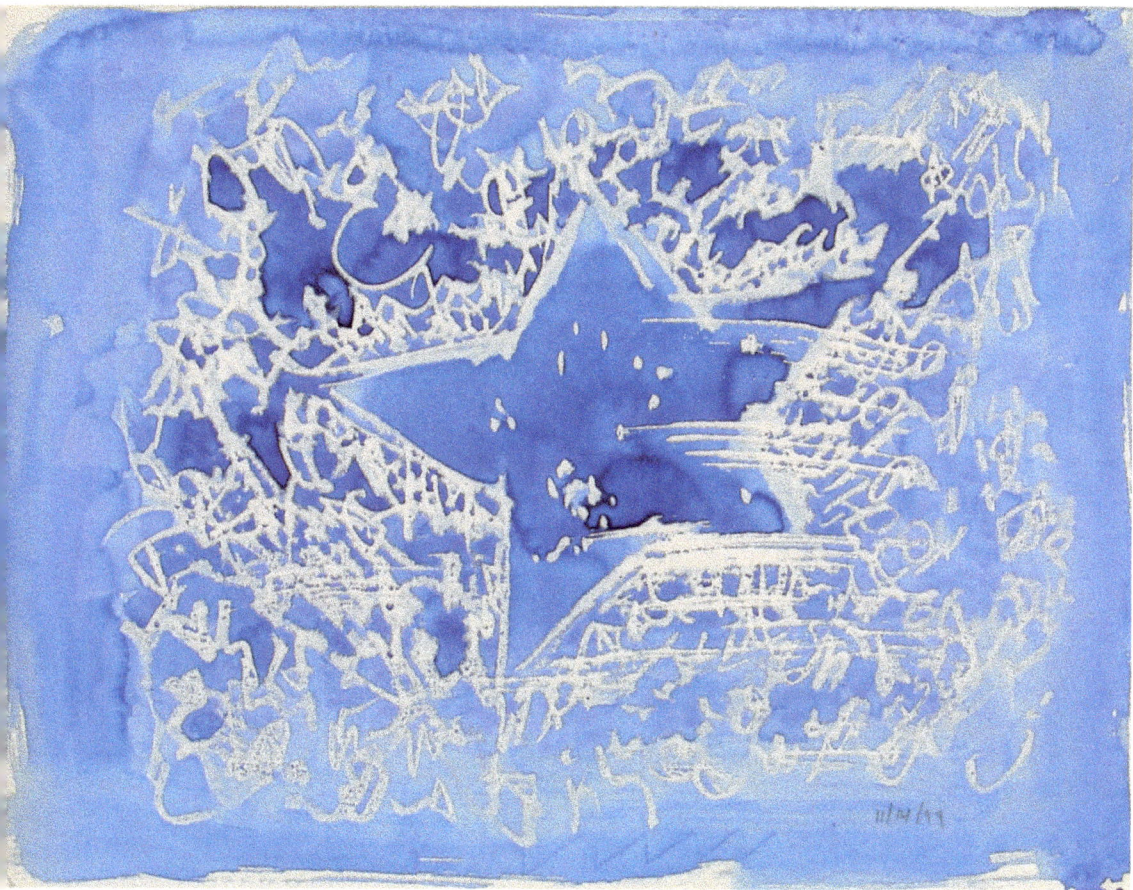

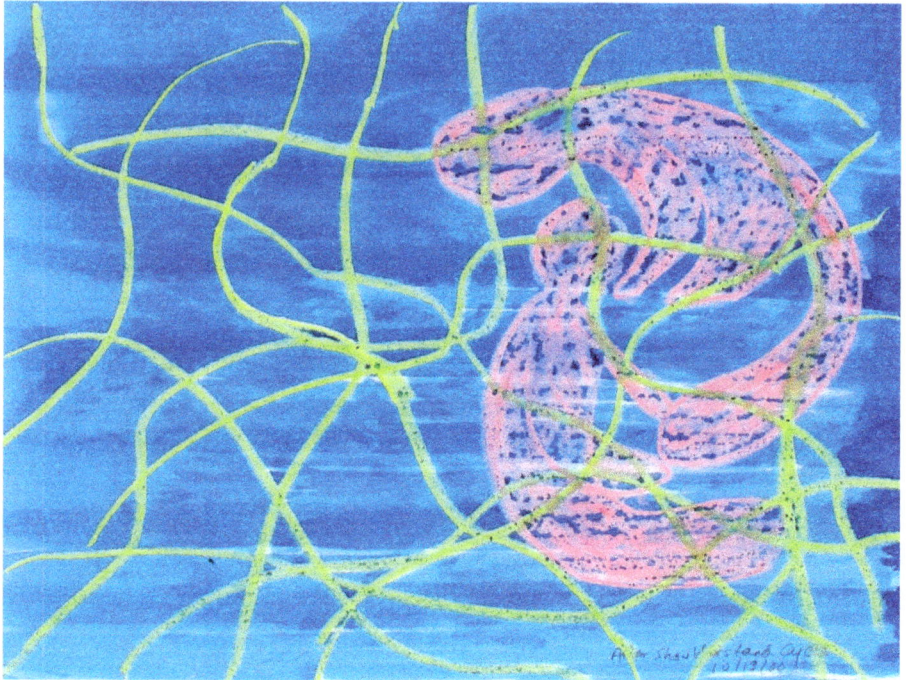

*I see clearly that the love I send to people comes back as a direct connection with, a vision or realization of, the true nature of these individuals. Charles and Lewis are angels sent to earth to ease the suffering of others, beings of light. Susan is a strong bright tower, a beacon rising out of nowhere, lighting the world. Charles is neither fat, nor thin. In fact, his physical presence has little to do with who he truly is.*

*Inside each of us is a piece of the pure energy, joy and love that is God.*

*When we are very quiet or when we see something that is the perfect picture of itself, like a flower or a rock, we see God.*

*Some people like to put a face or a name on god and say that god is outside themselves, different from themselves, and that is ok for them.*

*I say god is in each of us and so we are more than we seem.*

*We too, like the flower and the rock, are at any moment, perfect expressions of ourselves, but we are more complex. We have will. This means we can choose.*

*The part of me that is closest to God is my heart. When I choose to be awake in my heart, I am closer to God.*

*I feel my brotherhood with all things — men, women, animals, plants, and even the stars.*

*There is even a piece of God's pure light deep inside my belly and sometimes I can feel it or see it and these are special moments. I am with God directly and I know this is the love and joy that gave me my life in the first place.*

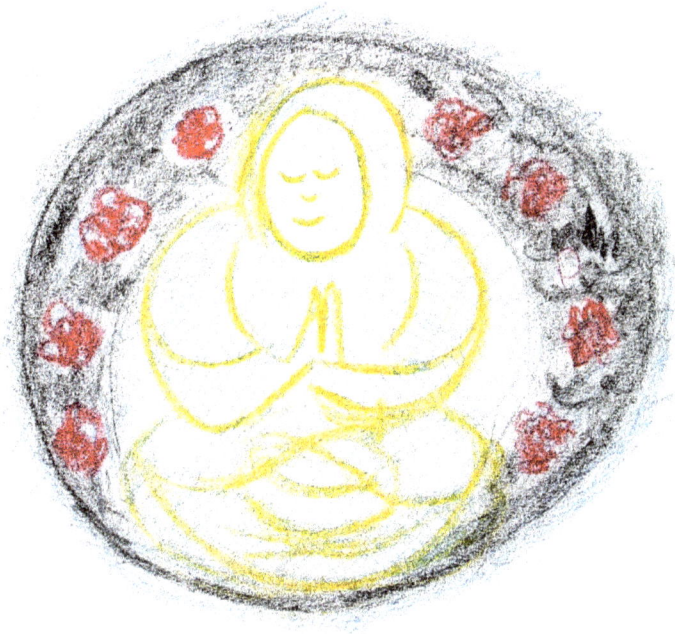

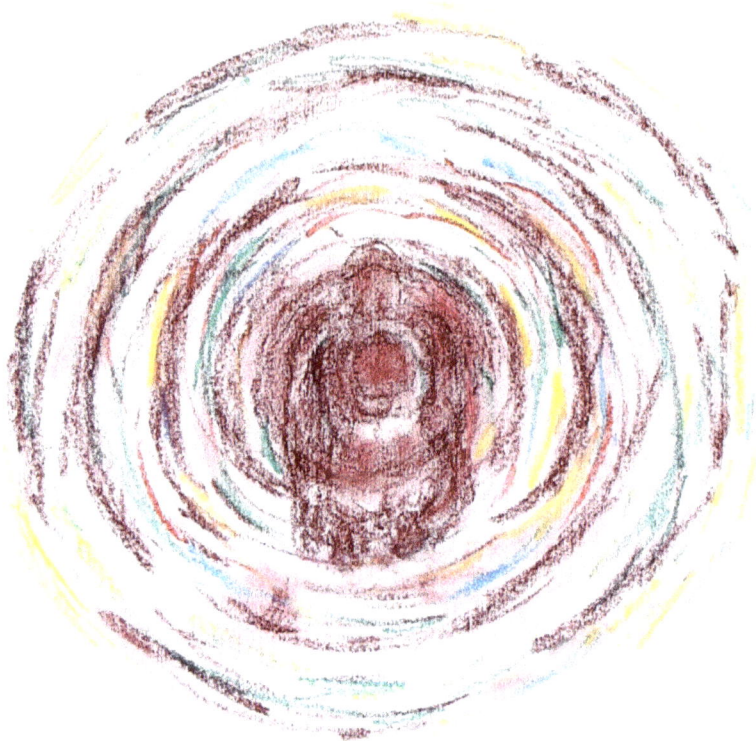

*The purpose of life*

*is to be the lamp.*

*To open the energy channels and*

*Let the light shine. I do this,*

*and I can do no greater service.*

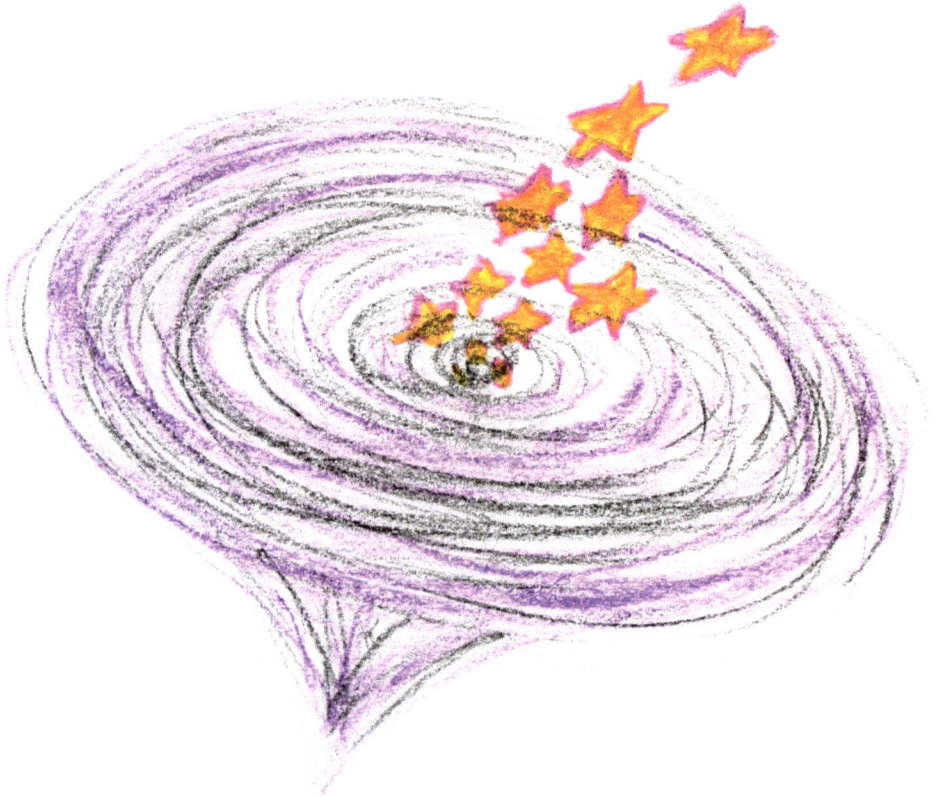

*Let go of fear.*

*Assume nothing.*

*You are capable of more*

*than you think.*

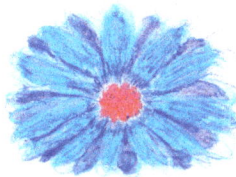

# Second Wave

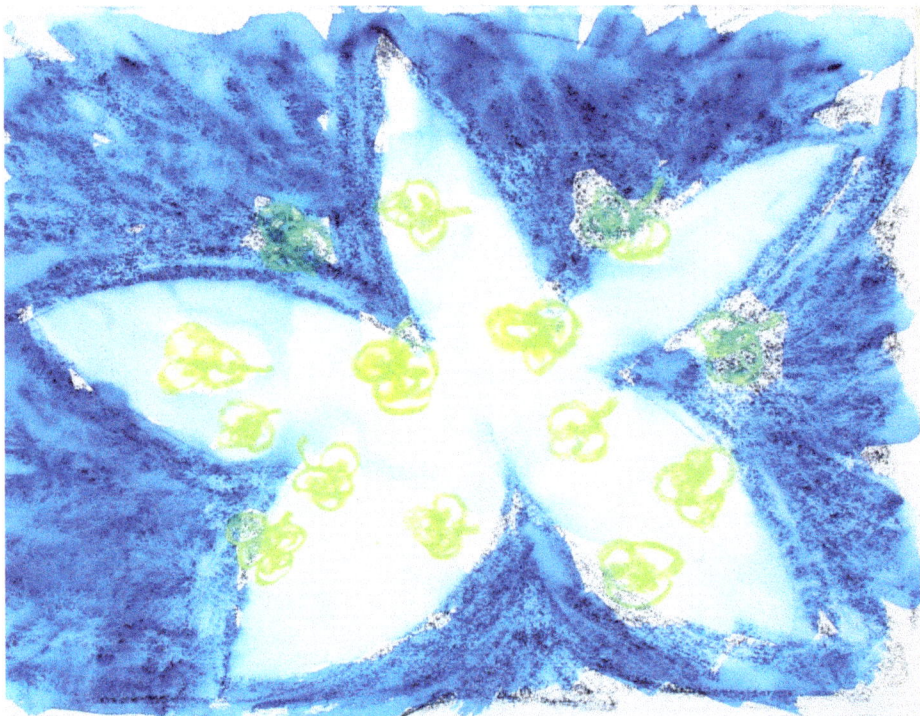

*It is Sunday morning. I feel closed off, stiff, looking for inspiration.*

*The sky is clear; the light and air are wonderful. My mind senses these,*

*yet inside, I remain untouched.*

*Now I am sitting. My back is softening, moving my eyes this way*

*and that, tilting my head, beginning to breathe. Listen! The birds are*

*screaming, the chimes are ringing. The sun is bright then dim as clouds*

*move cleanly across the sky.*

*I am not alone now. I am part of. I am inside and outside, together, as one.*

*Death asks me — What have I to complain about now? There is living*

*enough in this moment to have been alive for this once and only.*

*Today Death tells me —*
*This day, this moment is all I am surely given*
*and all I am capable of living right now.*
*I open my eyes to the light,*
*slanting through windowpanes,*
*my ears to the mockingbird,*
*and my heart to trust.*
*Worry vanishes.*

*I breathe deeply and smell the warm fragrance*
*of new, green life rising and old trees dying.*

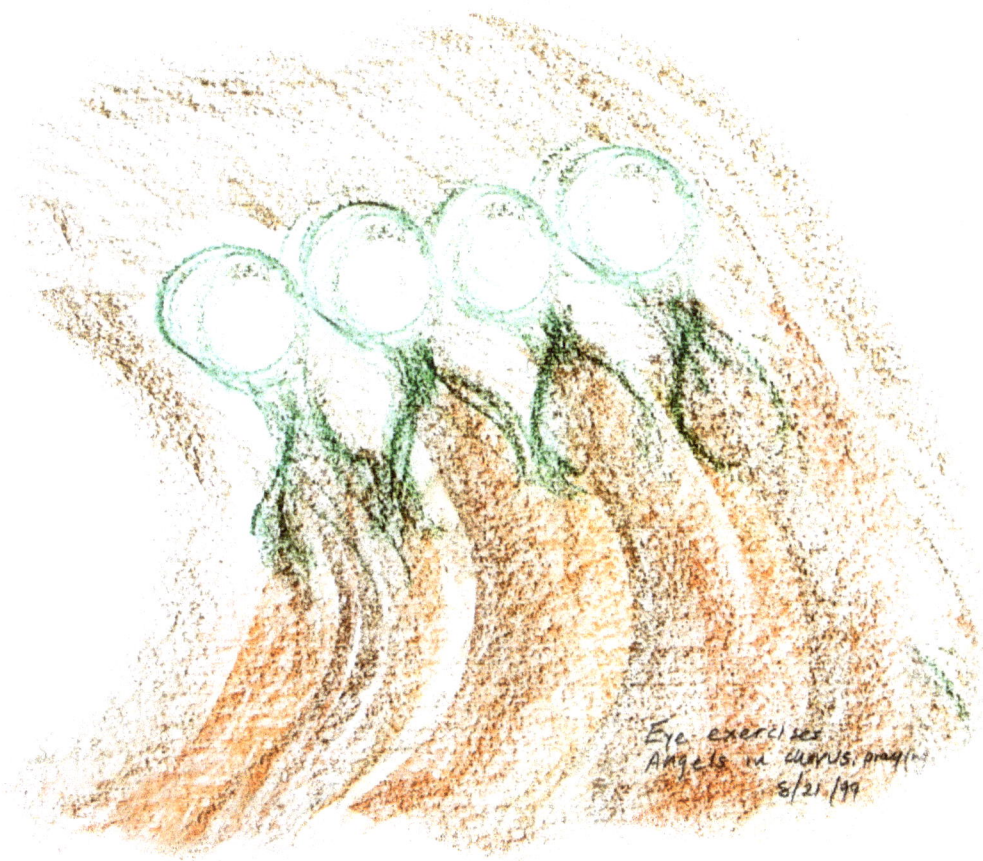

Eye exercises
Angels in cumus, paging
8/21/99

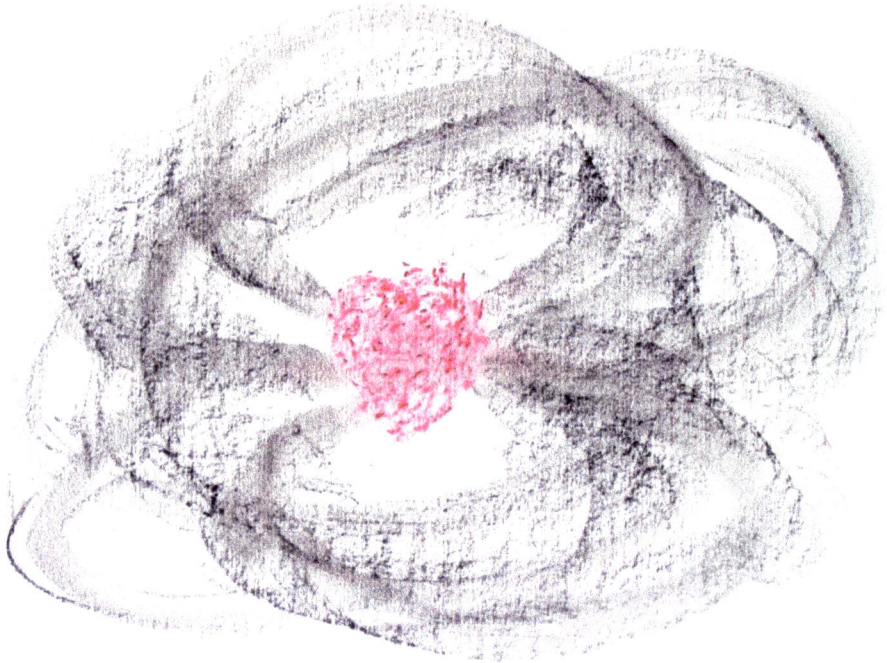

*After eye exercises, behind my eyelids,*

*The smoke of the incense of joy and gratitude is rising.*

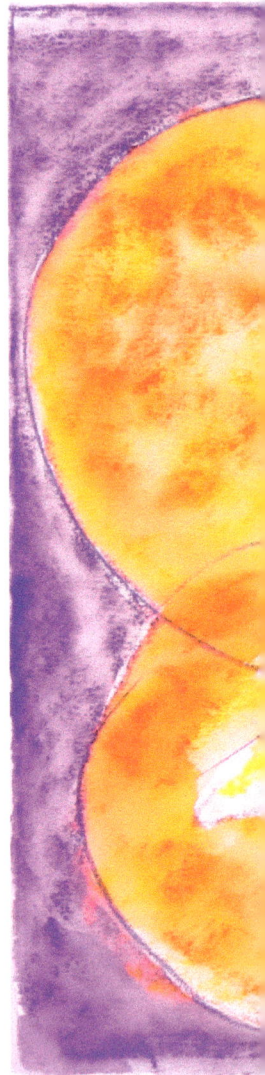

*After Twisting, there is a spaciousness inside my chest,*

*and sunrises in global skies, with smiles.*

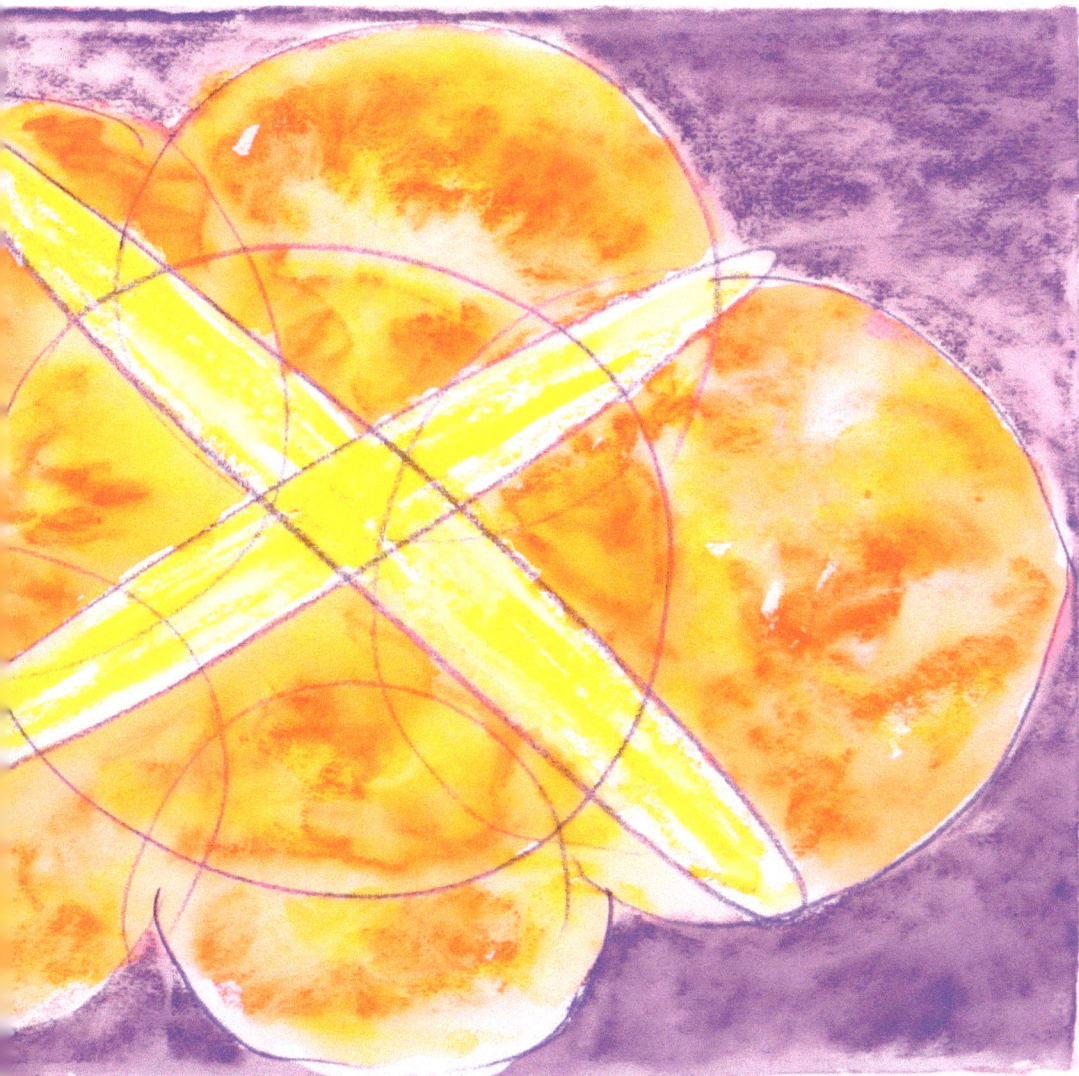

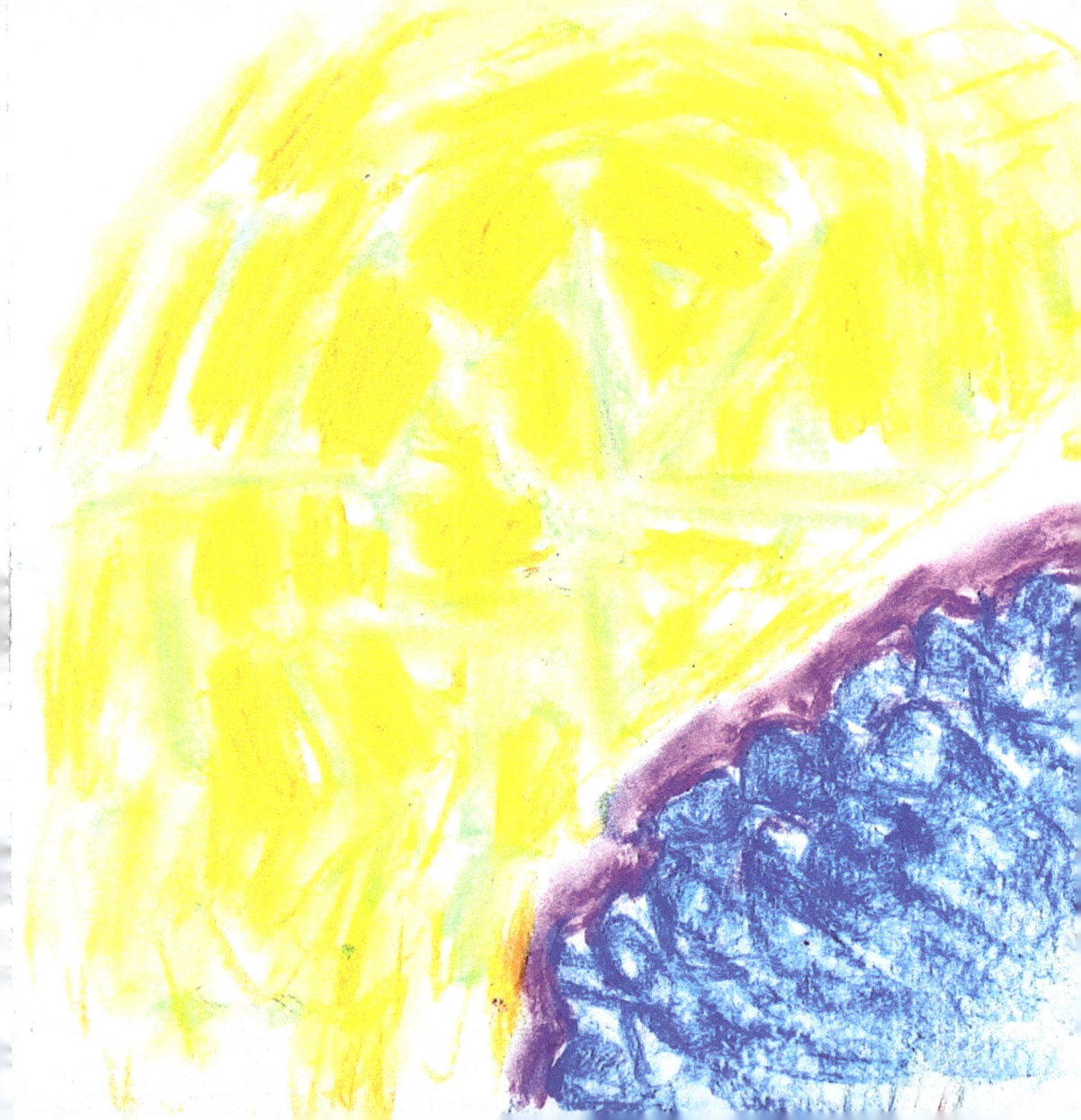

And I am flying over vast expanses of ocean

knowing that there is time to examine each of the

12 million swells one at a time, should I choose to.

*g before locust*
*/28/99*

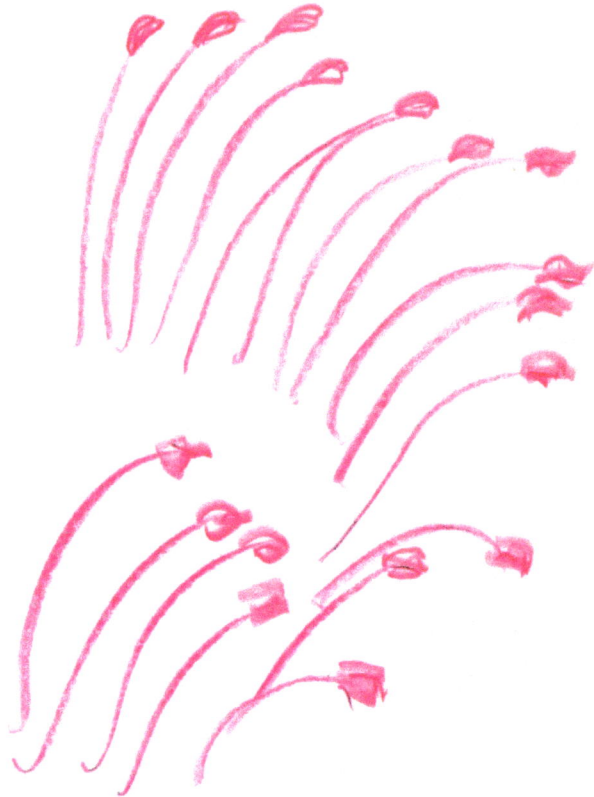

*This is the time that I am given,*

*each movement is the last and the first.*

*Sinking into the rest between,*

*moving again now, an innocent and graceful dance.*

*The in-between-times are really mini meditations; moments spent observing inner processing in body-mind-spirit. After Bow Pose I feel congestion clearing, and there are wonderful purple sea anemone floating and undulating below me in a sea of darkness.*

*R U S H I N G , , , , , ,,, I would have missed all that.*

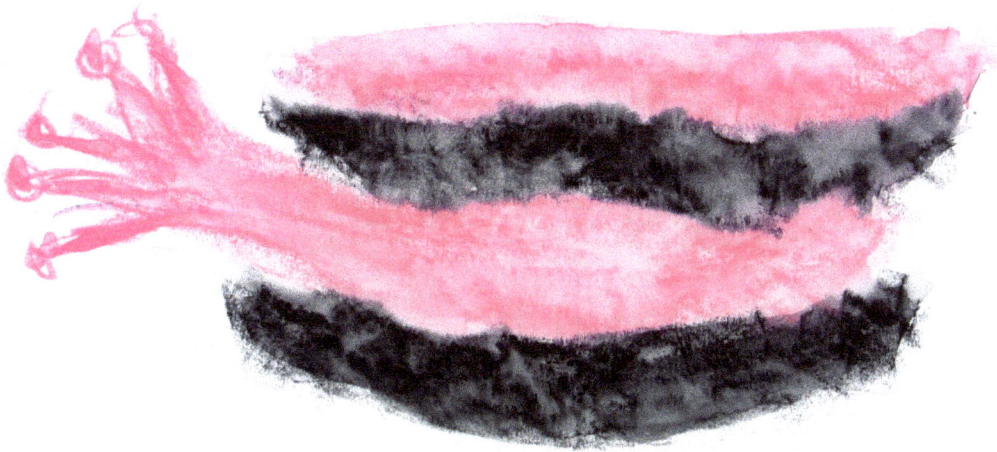

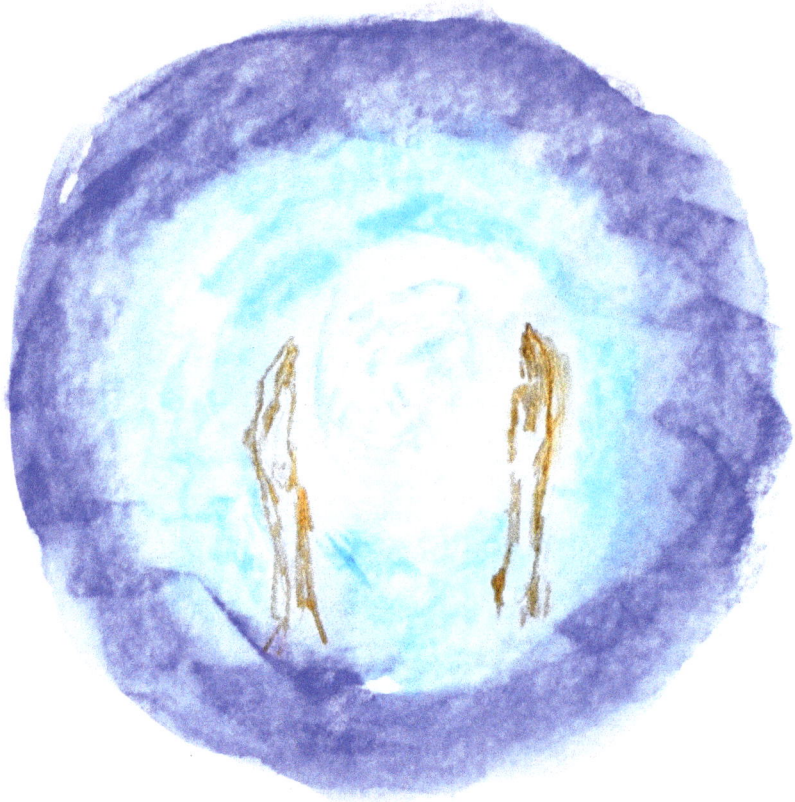

*I am listening.*

*Inside there is a part of me crying for some reason*
*I do not know… listening, I feel the pain.*

*Soon the crying place comes back to my heart,*
*and we are quiet and whole once again.*

*A lot of Learning is simply remembering things I already knew, perhaps in some new order or mode of expression. But what is Knowing? Knowing can change in an instant. The sense of Knowing can open up so wide in breadth, depth and scope, or hone into so tiny and gentle a space that the very concept or definition of Knowing changes completely. Each moment contains the possibility for infinite discovery; or else, the discovery of infinite possibility.*

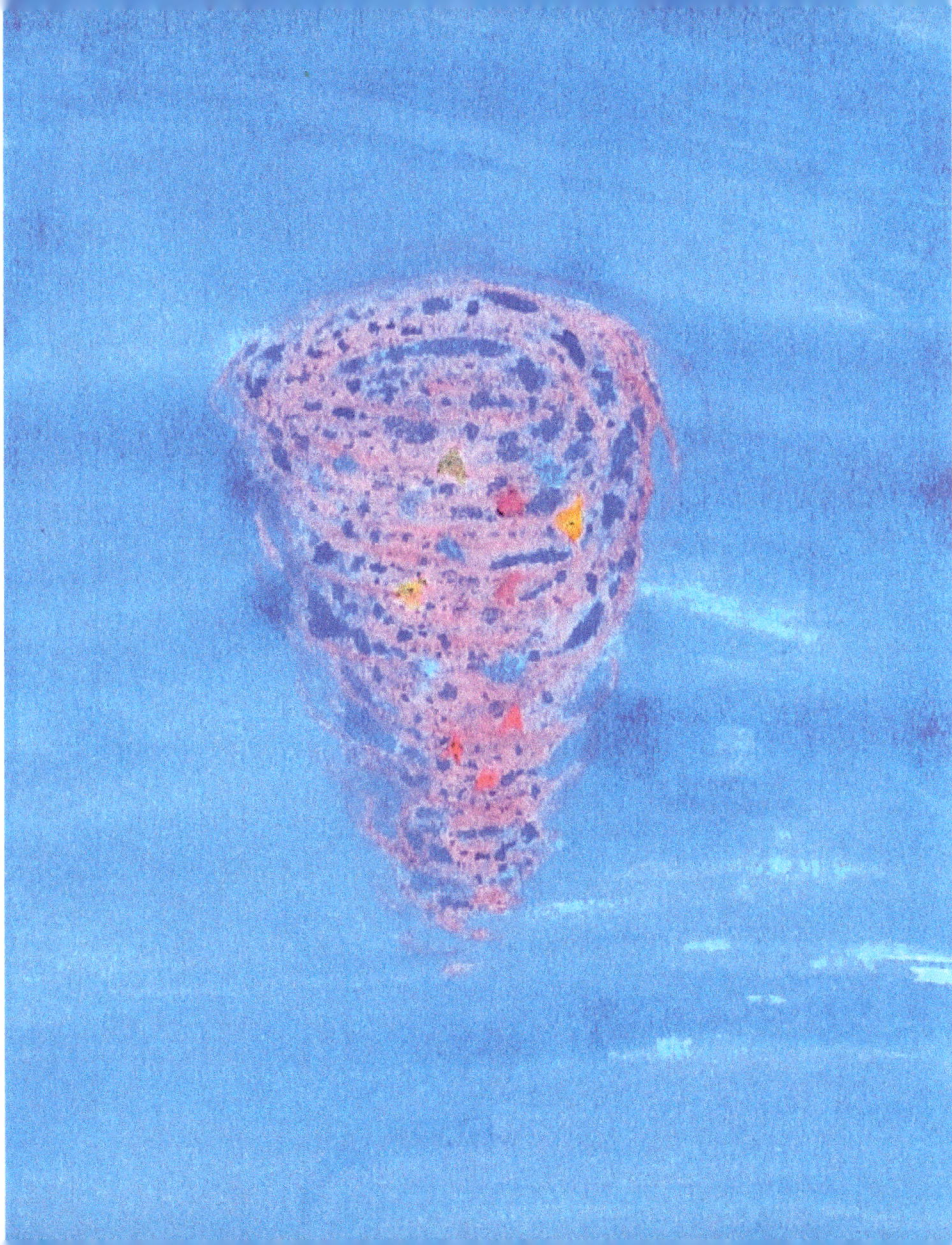

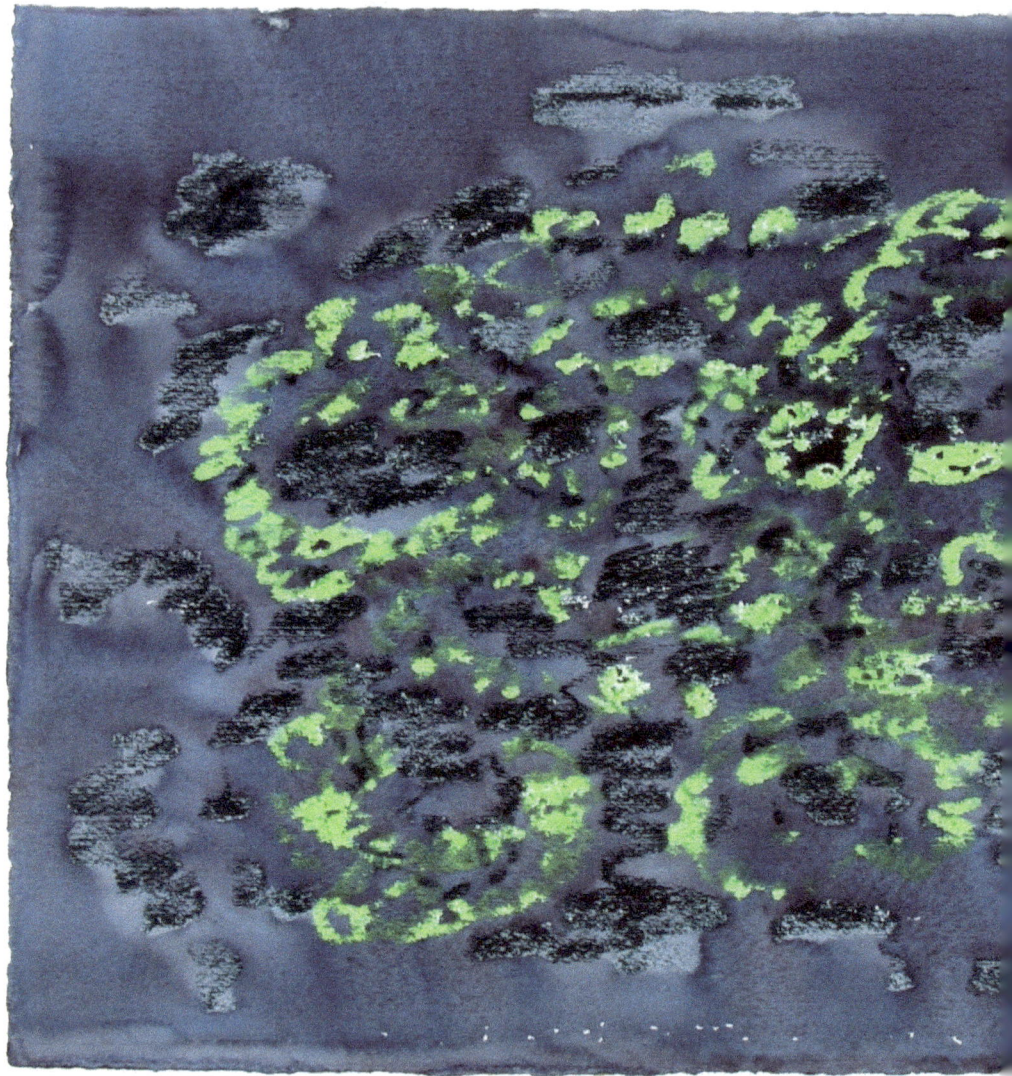

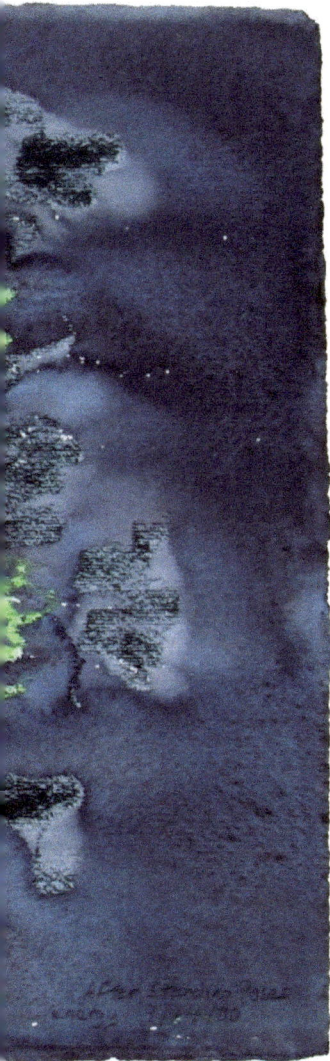

And I am floating in a vast richness of possibilities,
travelling on my own column of free-flowing air,
sitting apart, yet a part of everything. There is a place
where a piece of every thing and every one resides,
touches — some call it the void.

And when I open my eyes,
each object I have looked at so many times,
I now see more of, feel the history,
the makers and weavers, the vibrant, true colors.
Objects alive! — pulsing with energy,
multidimensional —
as am I.

Energy emanates from the handmade rug
my foot rests upon, all the careful work of the knotters
and designers. I am so moved — I am kneeling...

Even now, as I write, colors relax, surfaces solidify and
objects resume their more mundane aspect.

Easier to go about my business, yet
if I stop a moment and watch, listening,
I can still feel the vibration of their aliveness.
They only wait —
for me.

*I am a gift I have been given.*

*The more I let go, the more I am given.*

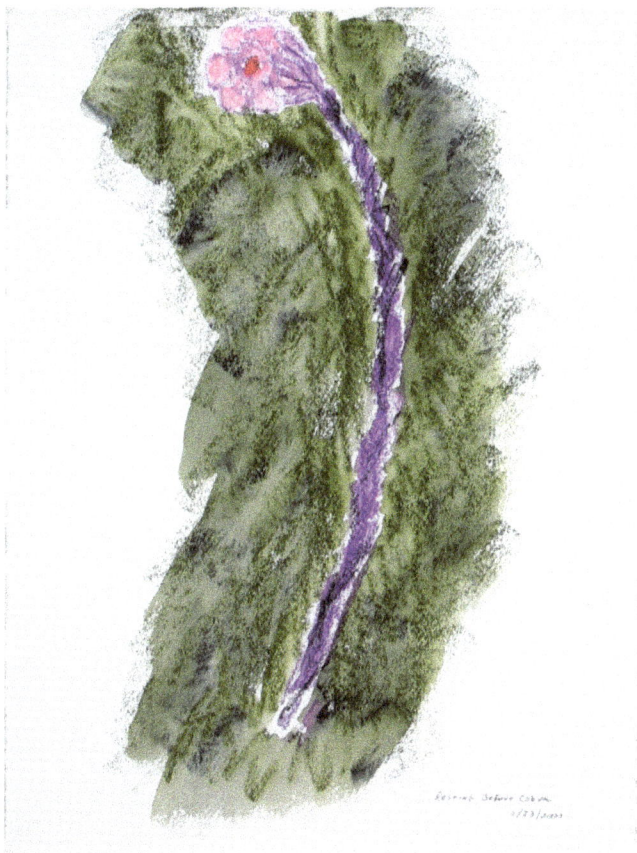

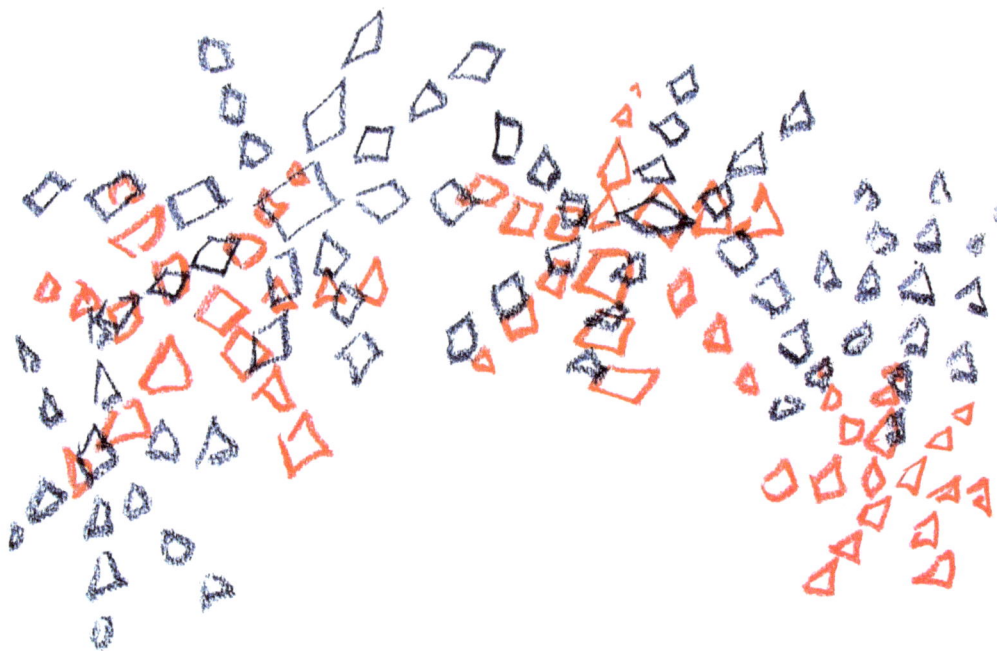

During Cobra 2/2/00

*Death is laughing at me because I refuse to allow joy inside me. Instead I yield another precious moment, day, week, month, or year, to stubbornness, robbing myself and others of many wonderful moments. I shouldn't think to invite joy inside unless specific conditions are met.*

*What a blockhead!*

*I see now that I have been given gifts beyond all riches; the gift of song, for instance, and something to sing about. I sing of joy, hope, faith, trust and love. I have no more time for tantrums, but trust in the purpose for this moment and all that may follow, listening for joy's arrival and giving her a lift on her way toward filling the world with love.*

*I give thanks to my spirit guide, mate and wife, MG for her love, trust and goodness. Without her I might never have heard my own song; might never have listened. I give thanks for my wife who has helped me to be able to listen, and hereby rededicate myself to listen always, in each and every moment, for the twinkling chime of joy.*

*I could say,*

*"I would love to have been ready sooner,"*

*but it does not matter*

*because now is everything.*

*The iris blooms now because it is ready now.*

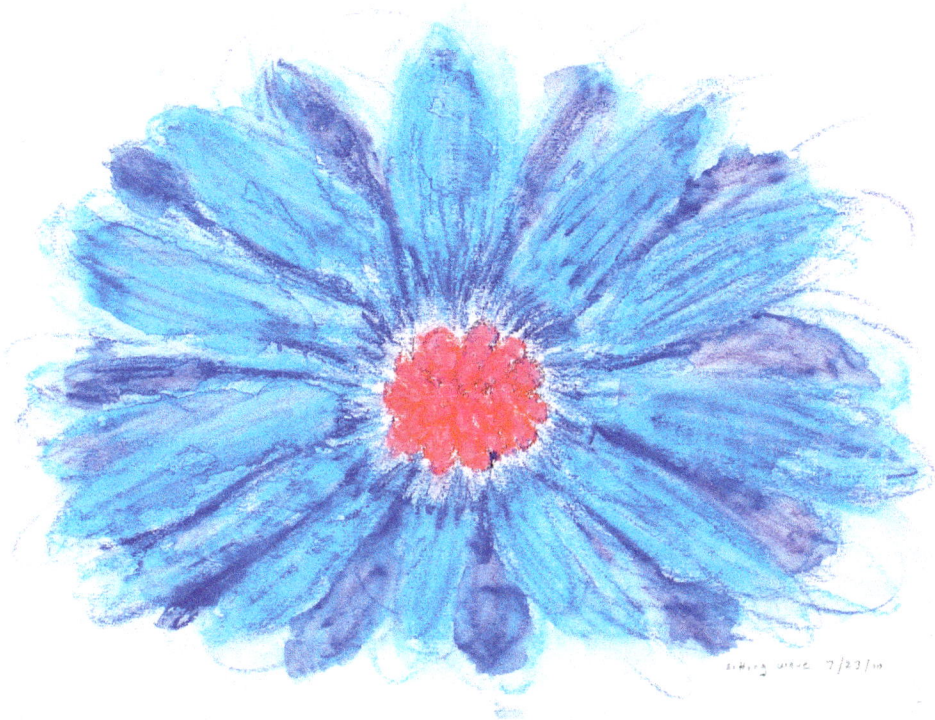

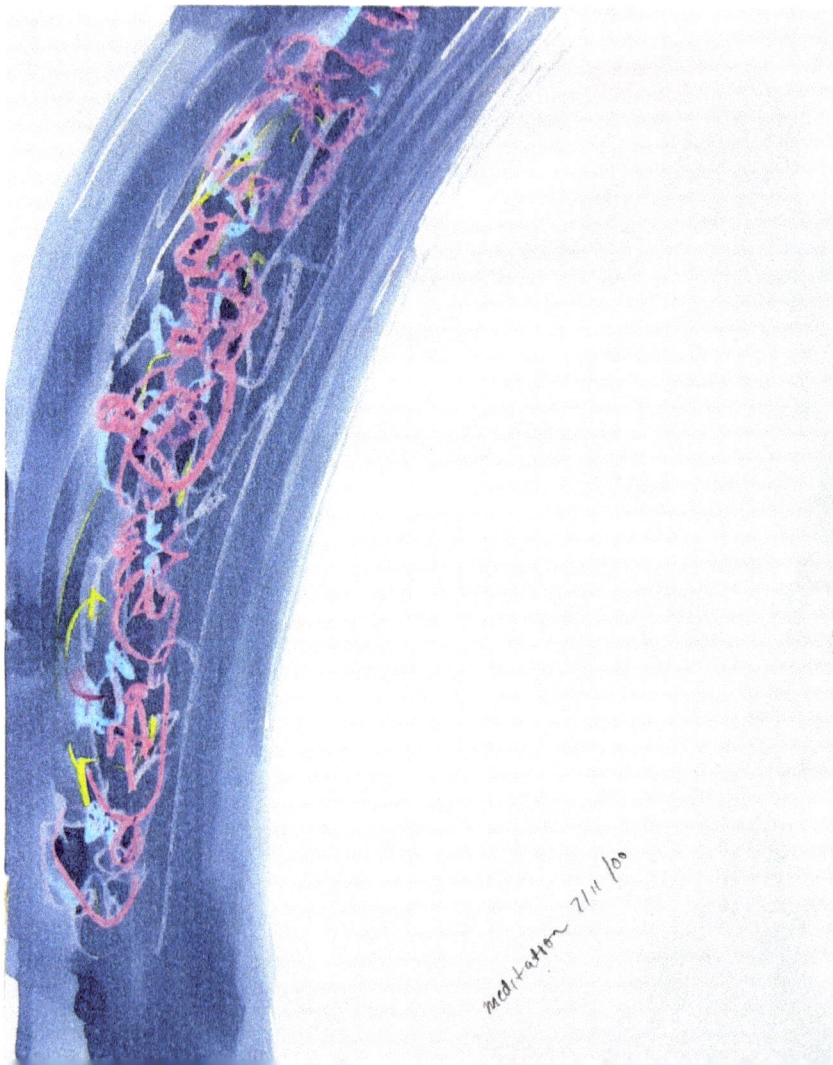

meditation 7/11/00

*Like a balloon on a string I am guided ever so gently,*

*solely by the breath. Letting go, I am moved and*

*straightened; the energy, lighter than air, fills me softly,*

*flowing up, through and out, effortlessly.*

*My heart fills gently, sending love energy to others,*

*to myself, and to my wife. Then: just being. Quietly,*

*healingly being for a while in grateful, open, restful,*

*life-giving, tender connection with…*

*I am poised and lifting, still and quiet,*

*gazing out the window into the afterglow of a summer rain.*


*Gazing outward yet inward, the glow of sky and clouds*

*resonates in connection with the glow inside my chest.*

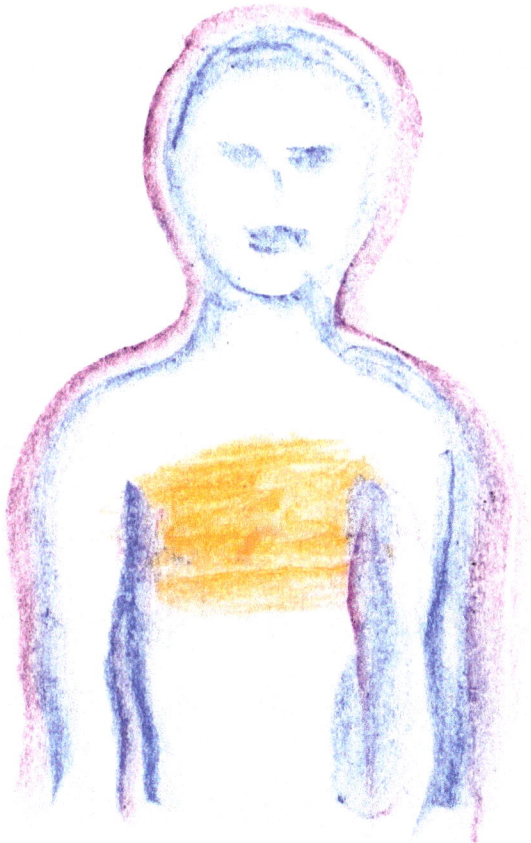

*Maybe I am experiencing one of the subtler bodies. It feels as though the weight of my physical body has disappeared, and whoosh, instantly I am in a new space. I am looking through a cloth, at first tightly woven, now infinitely sheer. Passing through it, or it through me, it is gone. Here, my physical body is no hindrance, almost non-existent, and I feel lightness, perhaps as light as the air itself. Certain patterns make themselves apparent, warm golds, and tans — energy. I have the sense that this space has always been here and that I have simply become aware of it, now, suddenly; experiencing, perhaps, a different layer of myself, and existence.*

*Energy enters the base of my spine and rises through each chakra,*

*enlightening, enlivening and opening the honeycomb of my energy being,*

*glowing like the embers of a good oak fire that has burned long*

*and is well tended.*


*Today the energy does not leave, but burns away Tamas and Karma and all*

*manner of junk and garbage, leaving me luminous, open inside my interstices,*

*warm and powerful. I send love energy to MG wishing her long and healthy*

*life; she gives so much.*


*I am sitting. Visions come and go. I watch for nothing, listen not.*

*Here is a bit of quiet, a taste of peace.*

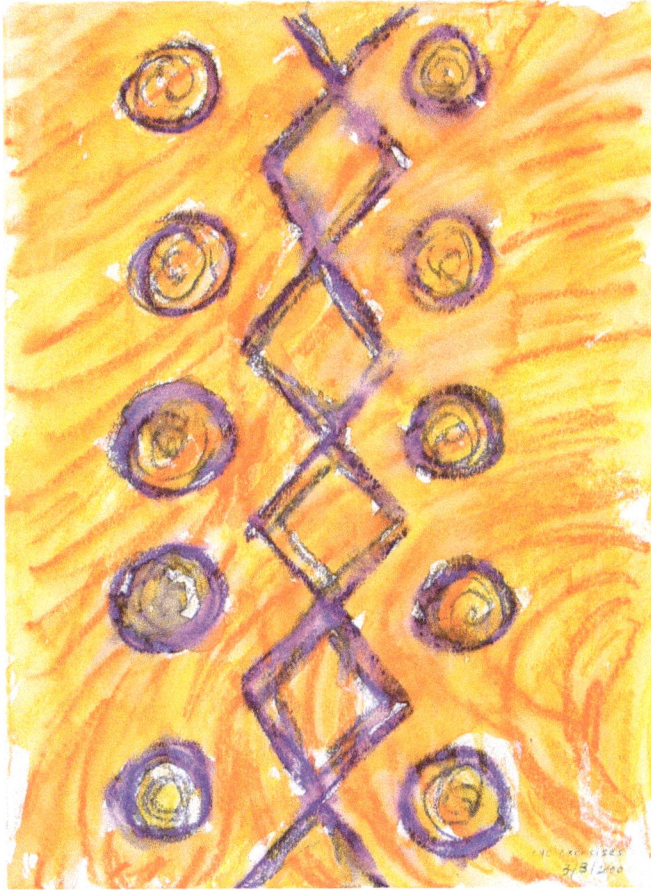

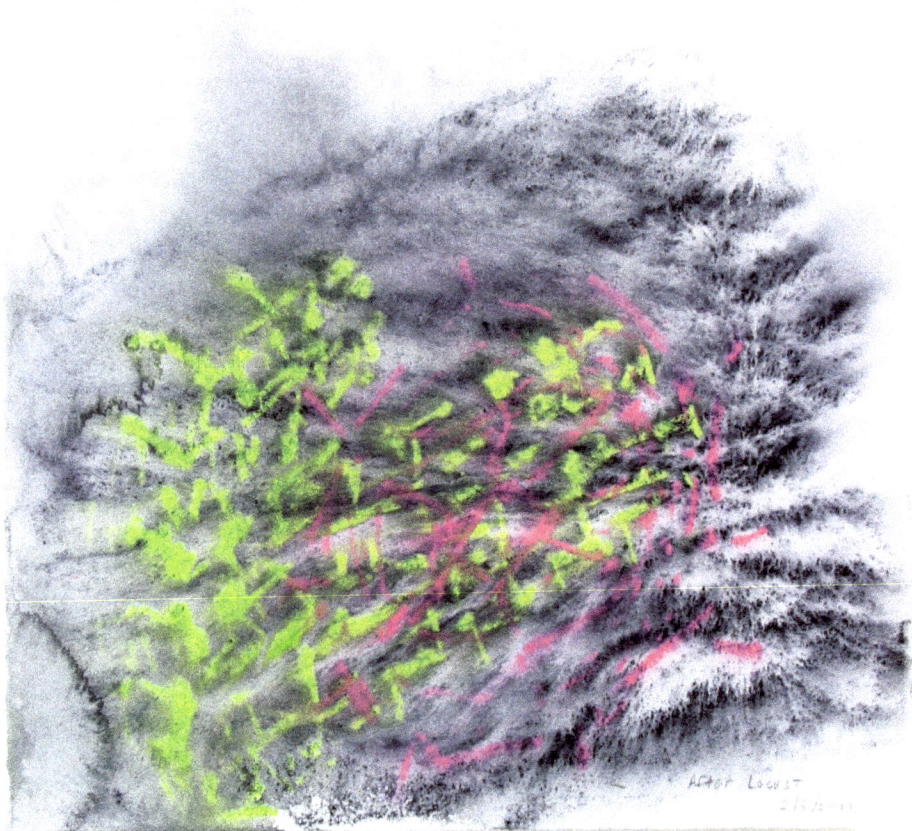

After Locust
2/5/...

# Inside Yoga

*The i that is me is here, but small; a sheet of paper dropped on the*

*surface of water, moistened and merging with other sheets of paper.*

*Not floating now, but suspended in space; expansive, rippling silk*

*of the soul, and my heart's core deep within it all.*

One wonderful peace is sufficient,

one moment of stillness,

in the presence of the All.


One step in the right direction,

once a conduit for love,

once a piece of the Infinite,

any one of these

is riches uncountable.

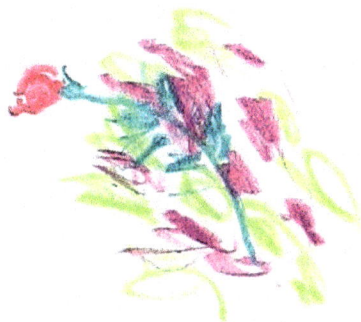

After Cobra
10/31/99

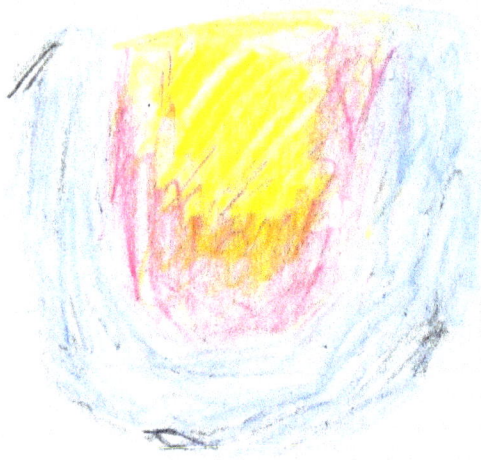

I am a cup filled with energy.
the cup, too, is energy.
(after Bow) 5/8/99

*A fulfilled life begins with the awareness*

*of possibilities and the experience of awareness.*


*Mind, body and "the experience of the infinite" are one;*

*all connected. The fuse can be lit from anywhere.*


*When body, mind and energy are united,*

*then life is full, and all things are possible.*

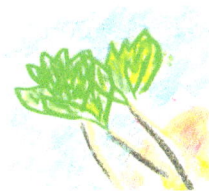

# Third Wave

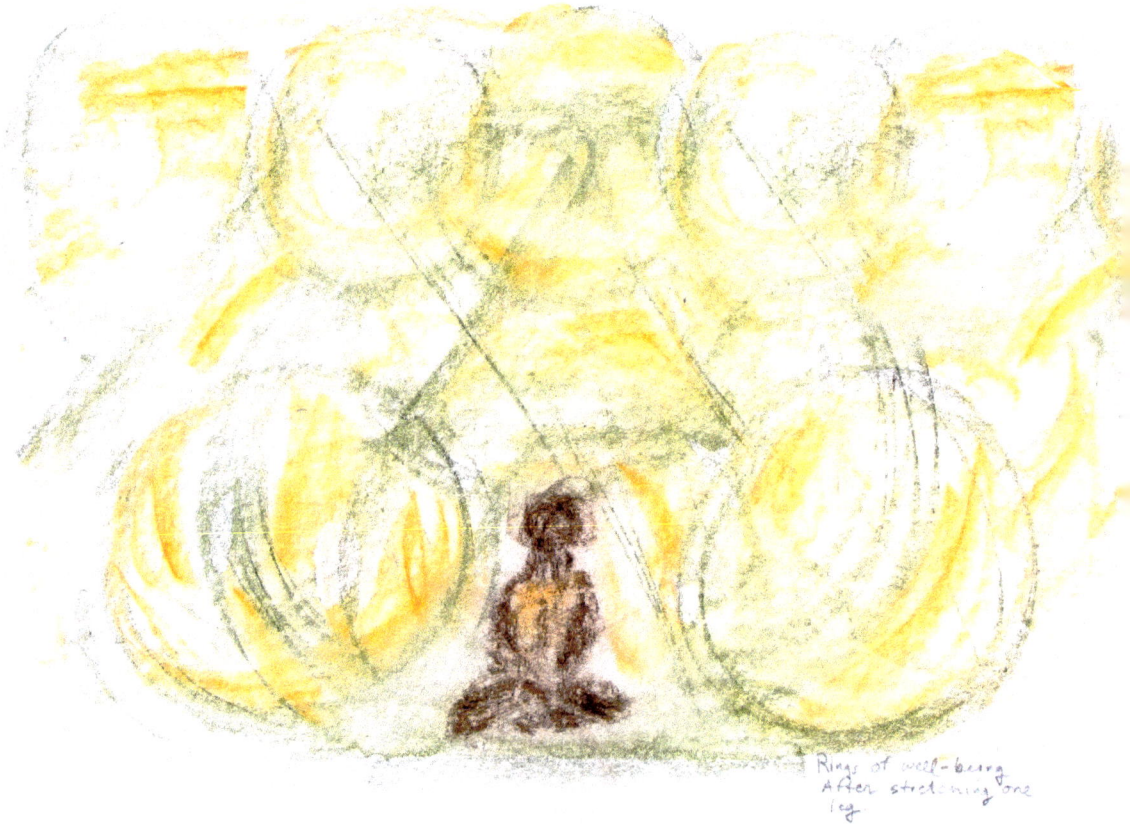

Rings of well-being
After stretching one
leg

*I go inside to see that which is vaster than all the worlds.*

*I go inside because it is easier to see me there.*

*But there is no inside or outside really,*

*Only the universe and me, and I am not exactly as I seem.*


*I am fuzzy and filmy,*

*Existing in many times and places simultaneously.*

*Big and small, a part of the All,*

*Grateful for the unlimited energy that is me.*

*I notice I am becoming small and spongy like a child,*

*firm, yet springy, like angel food cake,*

*but not empty like that cake.*

*There is a thrill inside me now that knows of death,*

*but does not fear, and delights*

*in long drinks from the welling springs of life.*

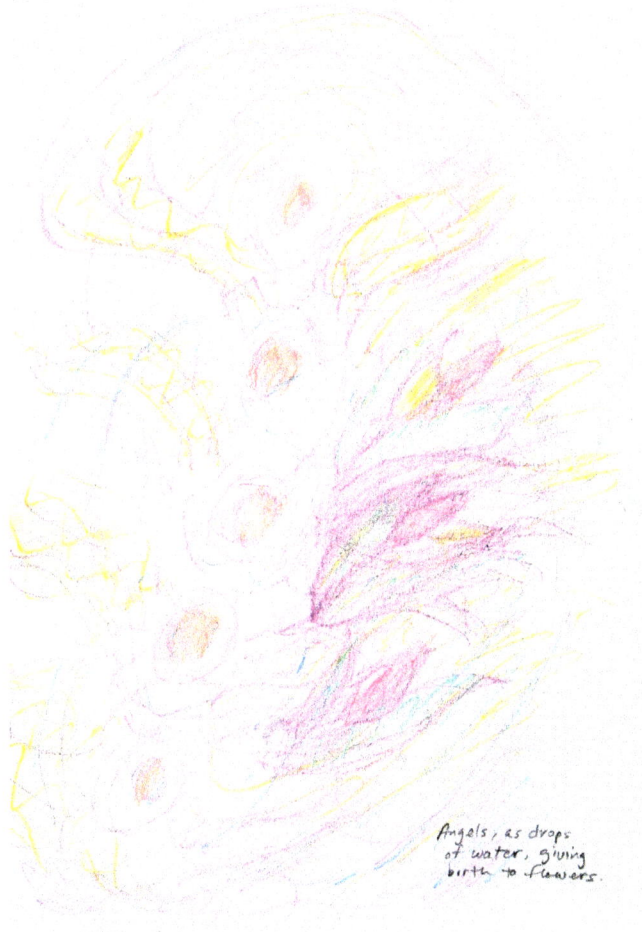

Angels, as drops
of water, giving
birth to flowers.

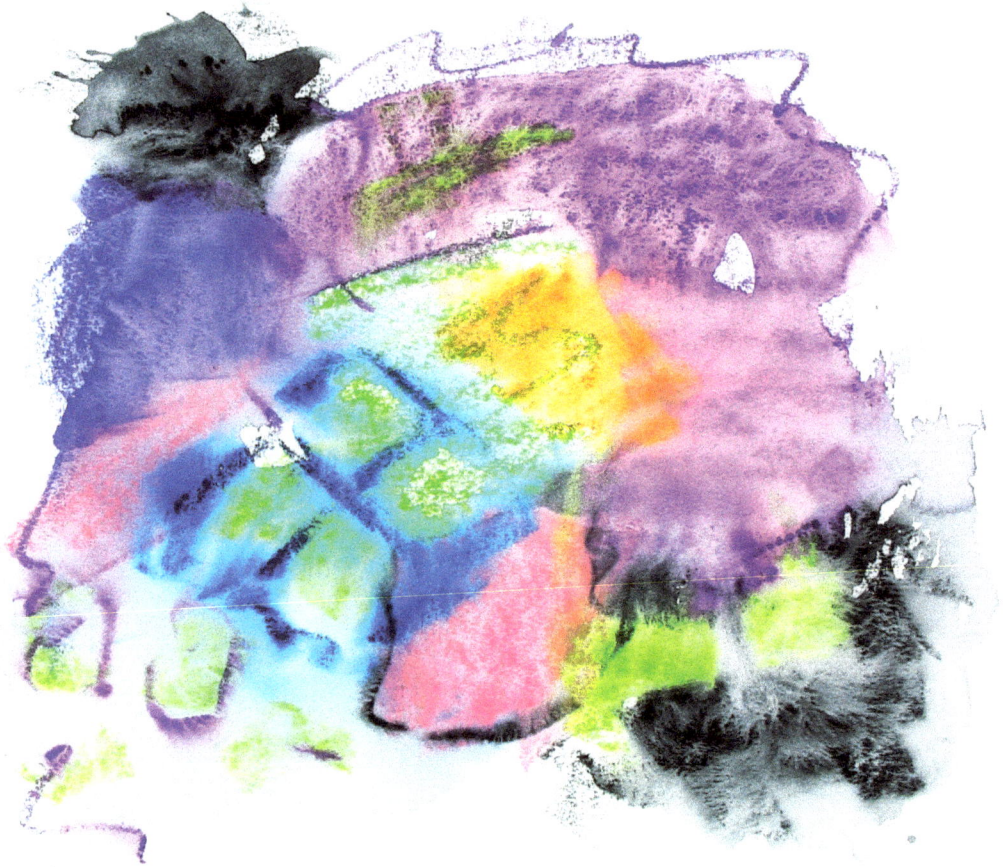

*The mind is like a chessboard that has been played to a stalemate.*

*Practice is a way of clearing the board regularly, watching new pieces grow in new places, with wonder and excitement.*

*Pieces come and go freely. New strategies are welcome.*
*Possibilities increase infinitely.*

*Each pose becomes its own world of power,*

*a lens through which energy is focussed,*

*a dispose-all for fear and restlessness,*

*clearing a path toward unity, oneness*

*and a direct experience of infinite potential.*

*The center is pure and clear,*

*shining like a brilliant light blue stone,*

*sending rays of light in all directions.*

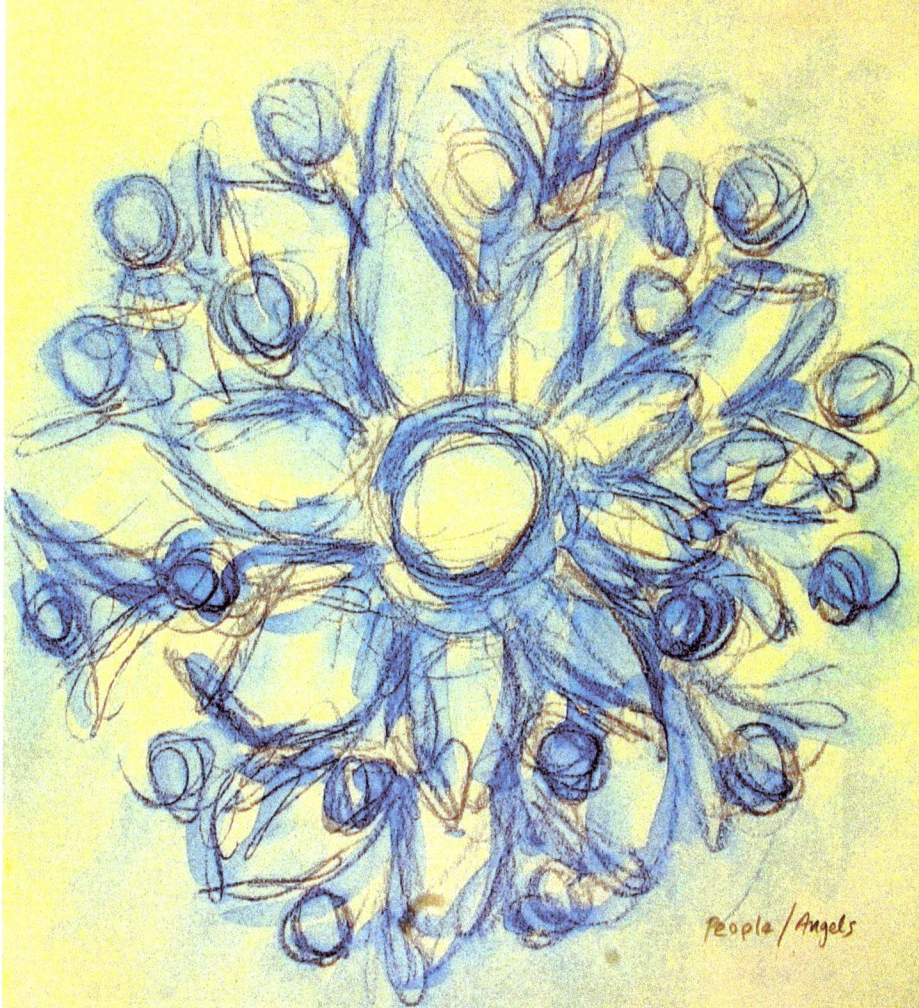

People/Angels

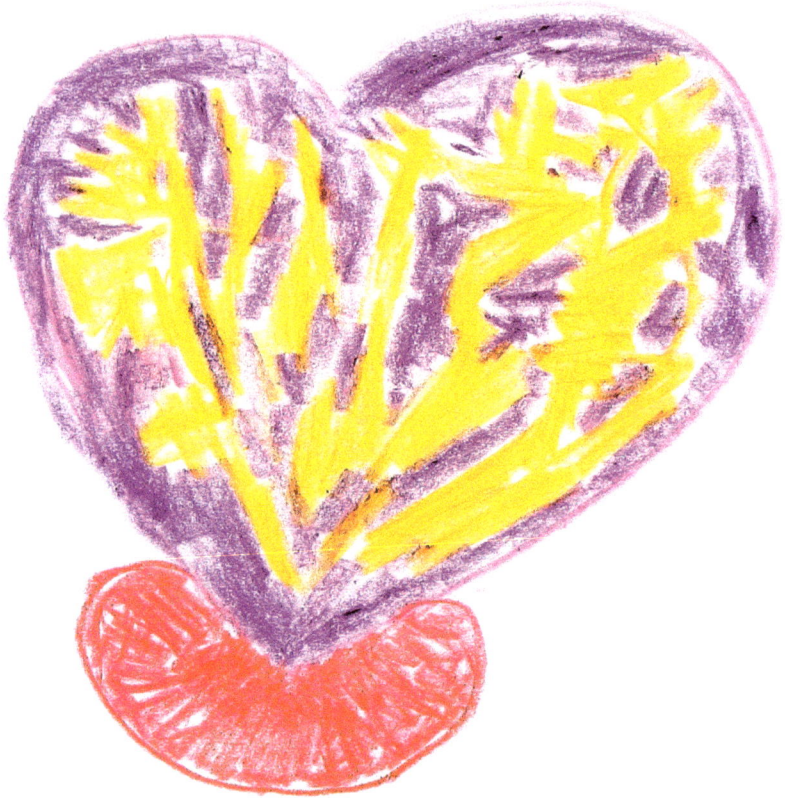

*I saw Vaz today in yoga class, Vaz's beauty.*

*Saw inside him, beyond skin, bone, muscle and tissue.*

*His beauty stood there, clearly present, as a matter of fact.*

*It stepped right out of his heart into the center of the room,*

*light and color beaming. I didn't question this at all.*

*The experience seemed quite real and true.*

*I go inside so that there will be no*
*separation between inside and outside.*


*It is perhaps ironic that I need to be alone and quiet*
*in order to experience my essential connectedness.*

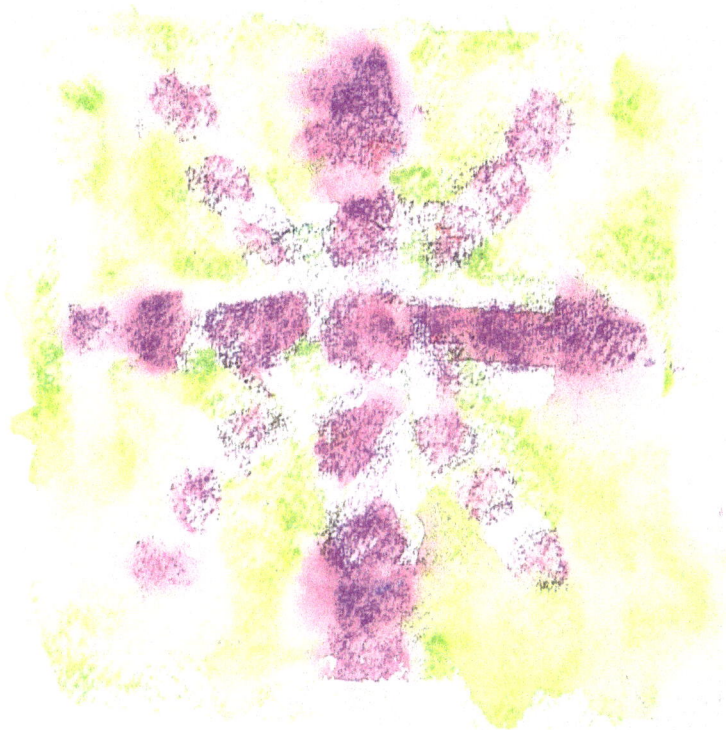

After Cobra

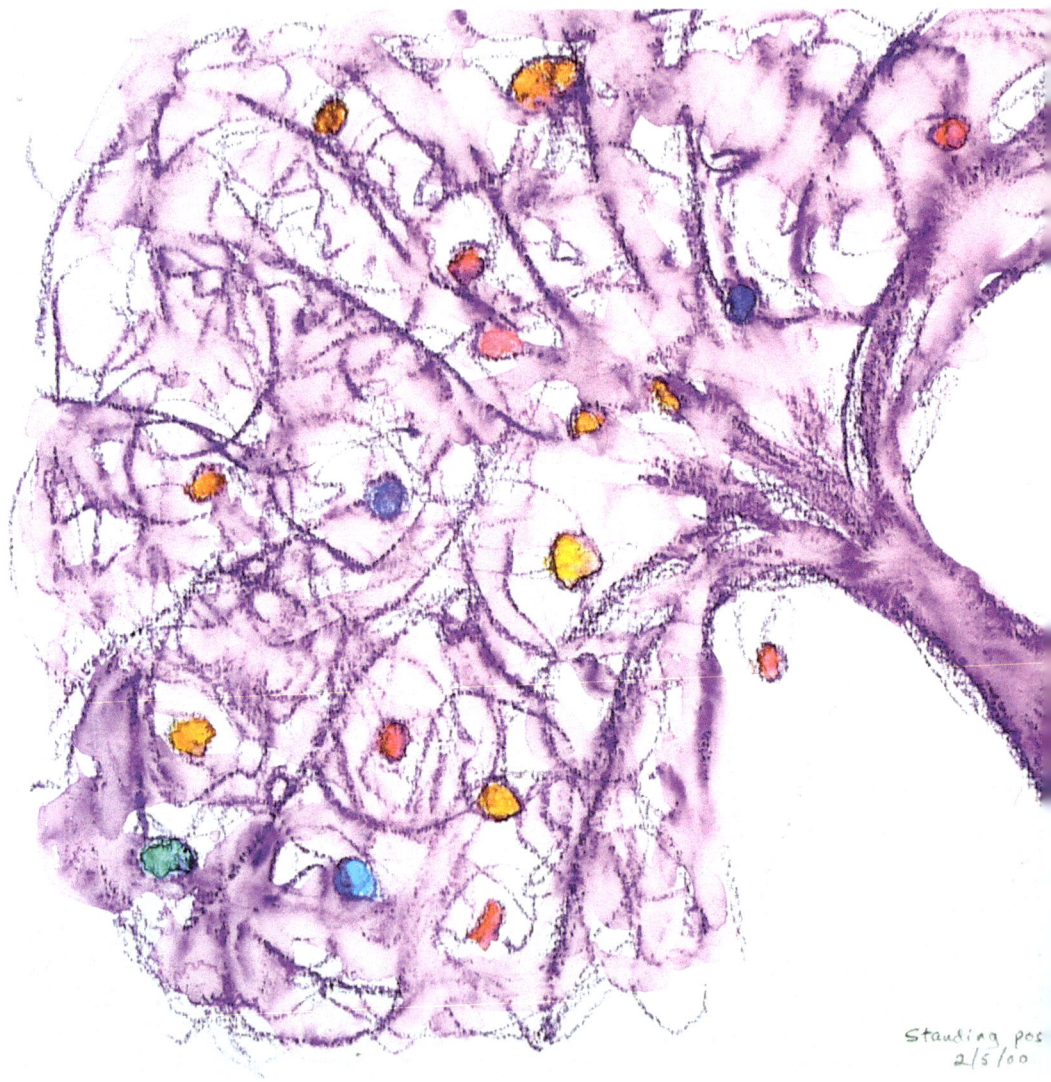

*Viewing the scene outside the window…*

*there is time.*

*I need not search to find the beauty. I do my practice.*

*When I am quiet enough, the beauty finds me.*

*I wear the clothing of compartmentalized life,*

*but here and now I sit enthroned in the fire,*

*wrapped in pink, scarlet and gold,*

*wreathed in the incense of dragon's smoke.*


*Crowned with the vastness of space, my heart*

*glows pink and red in my golden chest.*

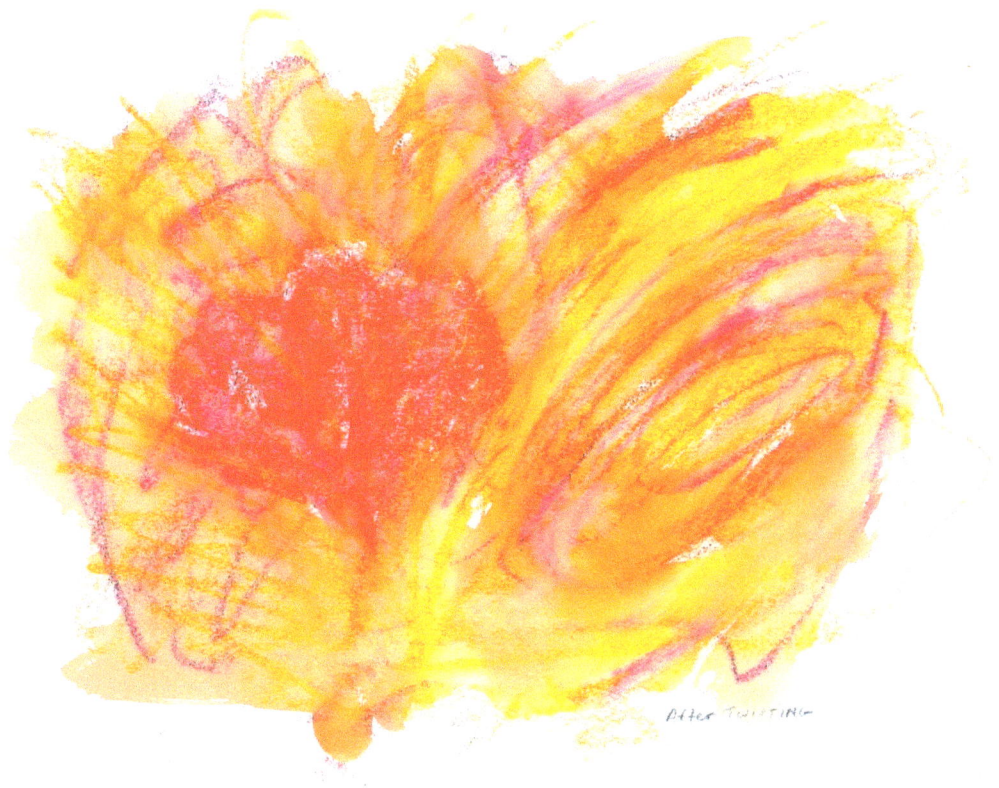

After Twisting

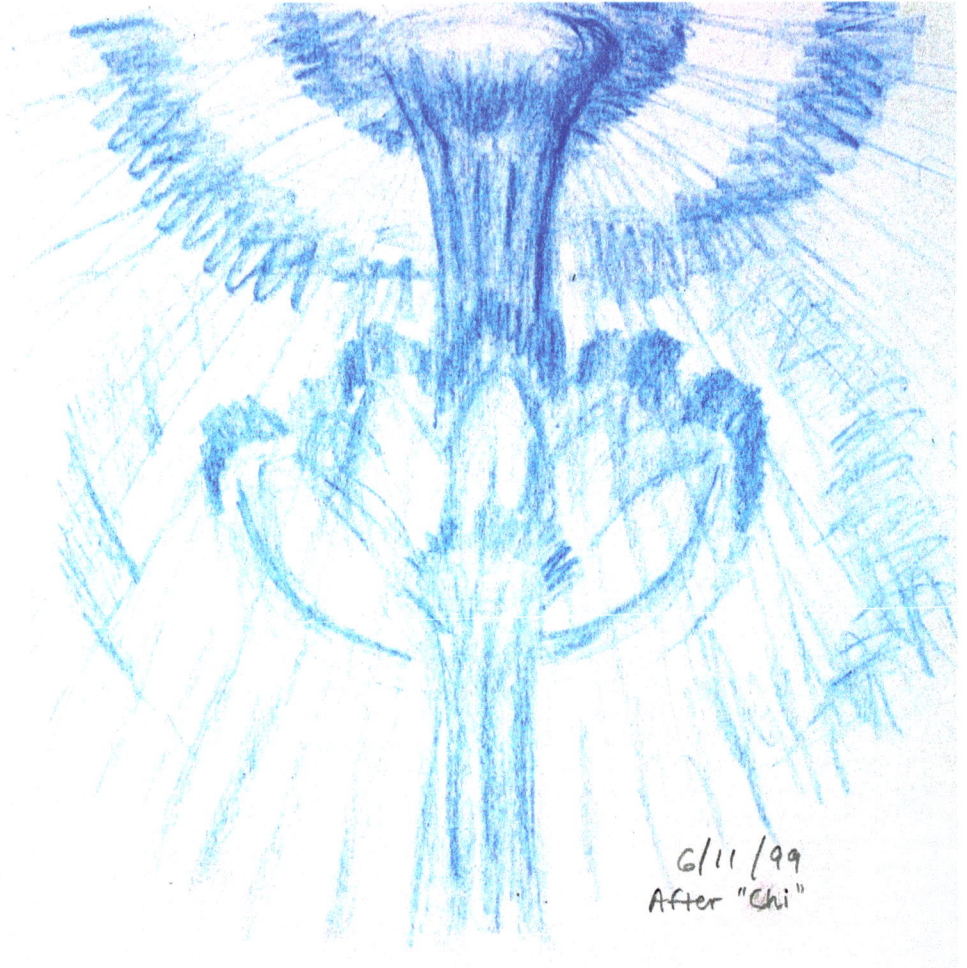

6/11/99
After "Chi"

*My energy conduit expands and*

*passes out through my skin.*

*I am transparent, spiritual organs visible*

*as flowers and symbols.*


*I am my energy body,*

*energy flowing into my heart, and out again*

*to all those whom my daily desires*

*brush up against, in this world of ours.*

*I am a diamond, strong, clear, supported and deeply quiet,*

*my lower back coming suddenly alive…*

*I am a flame or fragrant smoke wafting skyward,*

*a snake rising or a single flower growing toward the sun.*

*As soft as smoke and strong as diamond, another piece of me*

*has come home.*

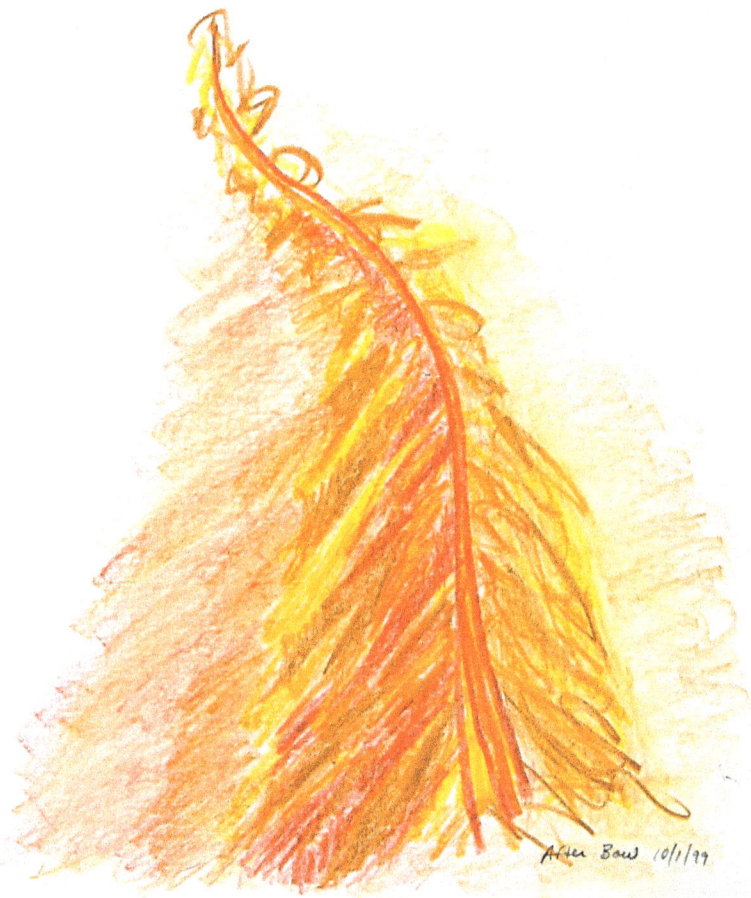

After Bow 10/1/99

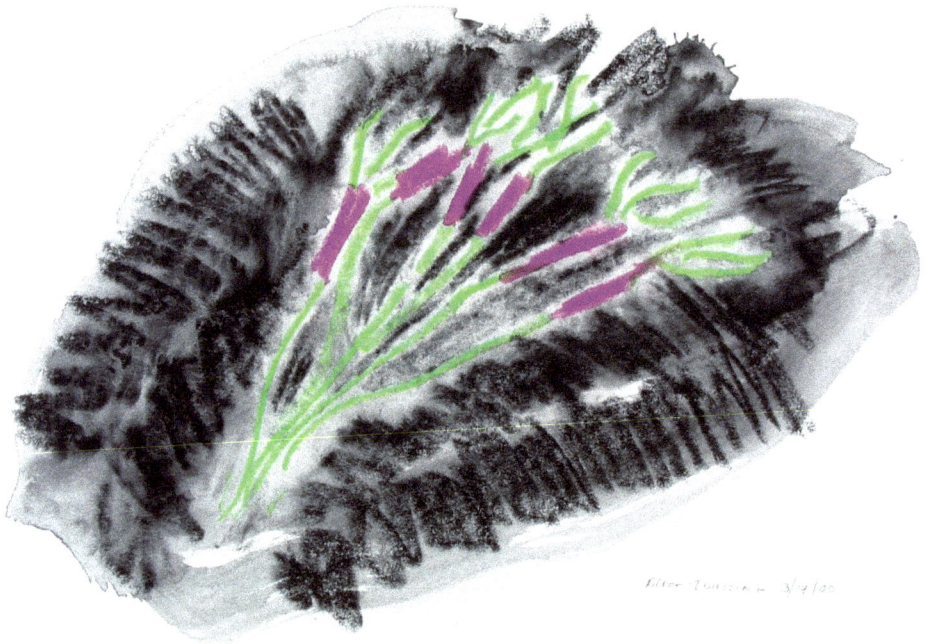

# *Inside Yoga*

*I am sitting in a quiet place,*

*inside the stillness,*

*shedding the skins of weeklong, headstrong antics.*

*I know I am forgiven, because I am here.*


*I come here to shed skin,*

*and to light the glow that shines through me,*

*as through a well pampered complexion,*

*so less stuff sticks to me when I*

*walk in the world.*

*Practicing Tree Pose, I focus my eye on some point outside the window.*

*Beyond that point my gaze turns a corner and comes back to me, finding a*

*quiet place inside my chest, energy flowing in and out, gently, continuously.*

*I am filled with lightness.*


*My foot grows phantom roots, down, into the ground, not to hold, but*

*to connect with the earth. Arms lift and reach gently skyward. I am*

*breathing lightly.*


*I practice this pose because I love it. As I finish, the two bookends of me*

*rejoin; a long liquid midline glued together in harmonious balance. I am*

*smiling slightly, involuntarily, catching myself gazing toward the trees outside.*

*The crepe myrtles are blooming, framing a gray-white sky.*

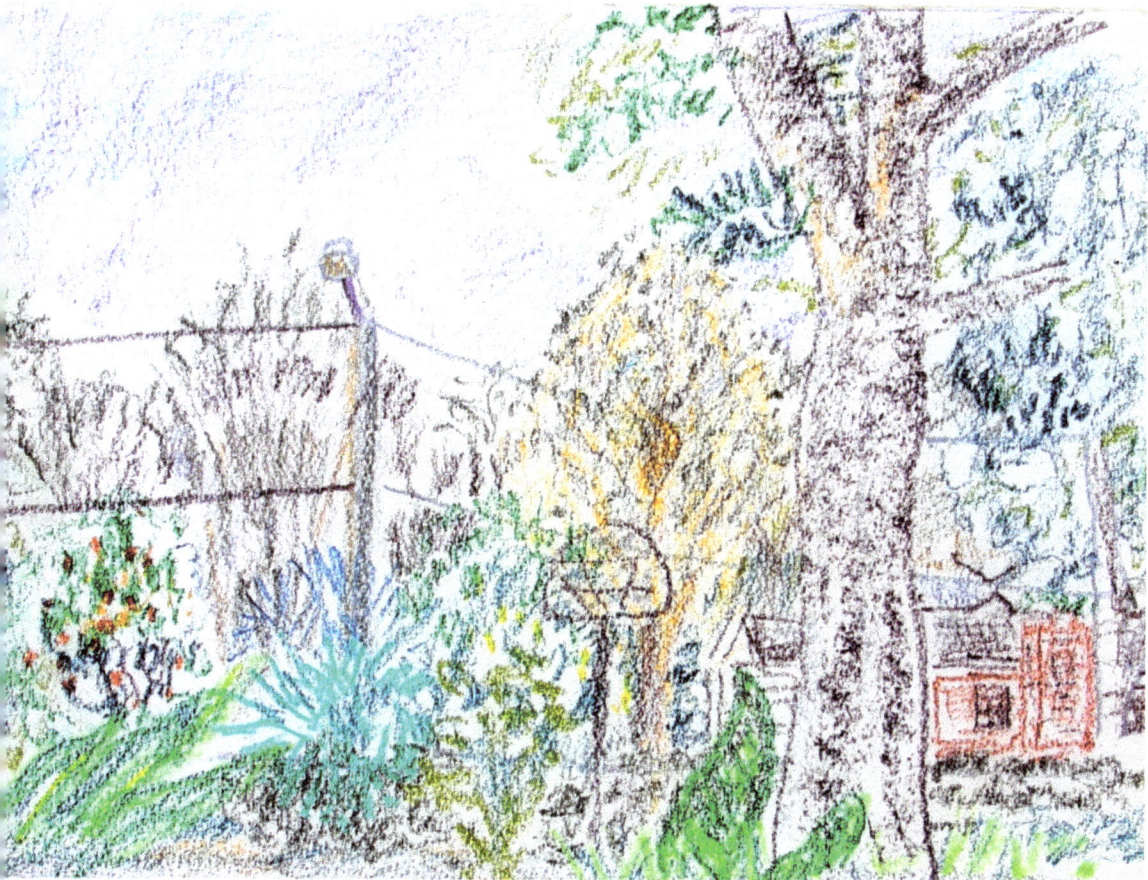

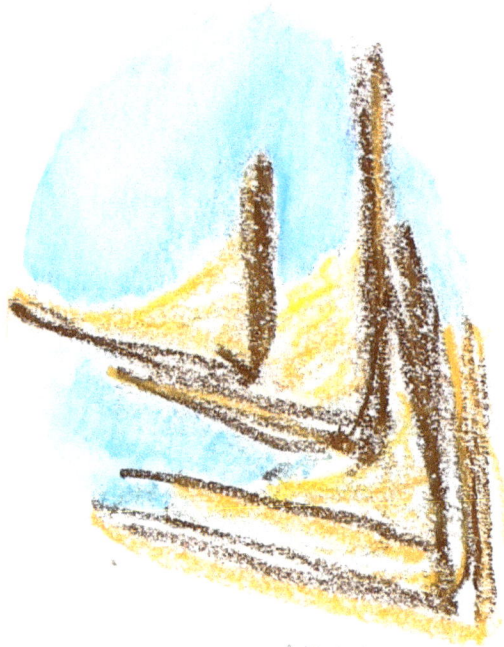

eye exercises
2/13/99

*As Tree my gaze travels out and in so that*

*two points resound and echo together;*

*a place beyond the tree perhaps,*

*a tiny patch of blue,*

*and inside me too.*

*Today would be a good day to die,*

*because I have lived!*

*I would not choose death because this life,*

*this consciousness,*

*is a greater gift than any imaginable.*

*Yet I do not fear death, because*

*I have lived.*

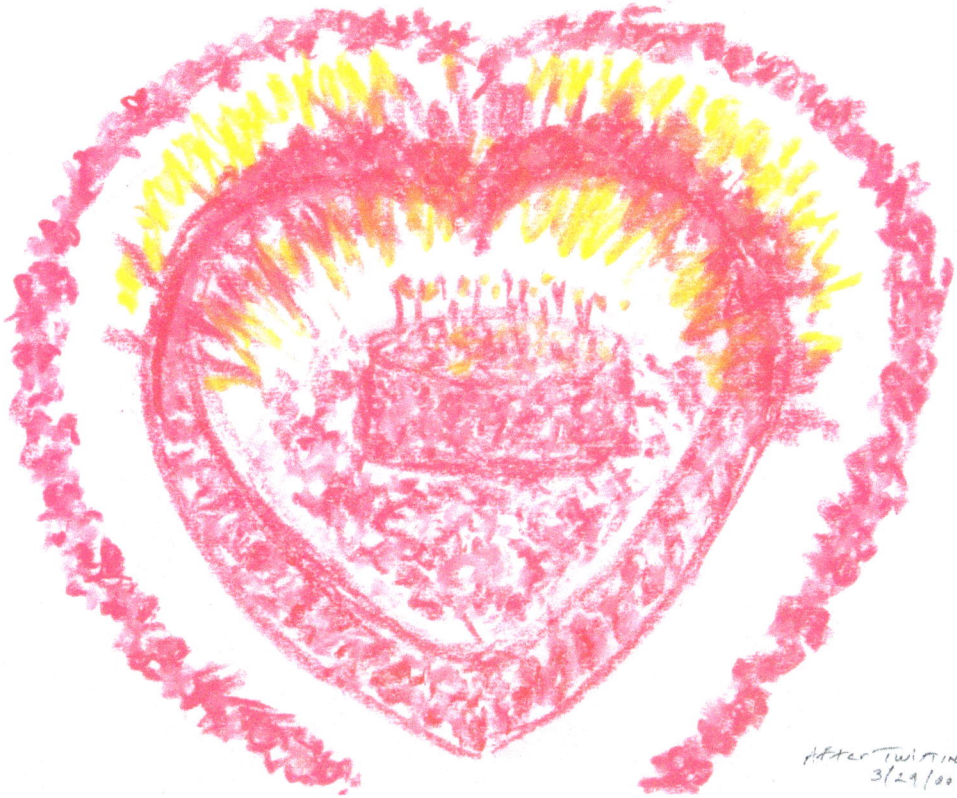

After Twisting
3/29/00

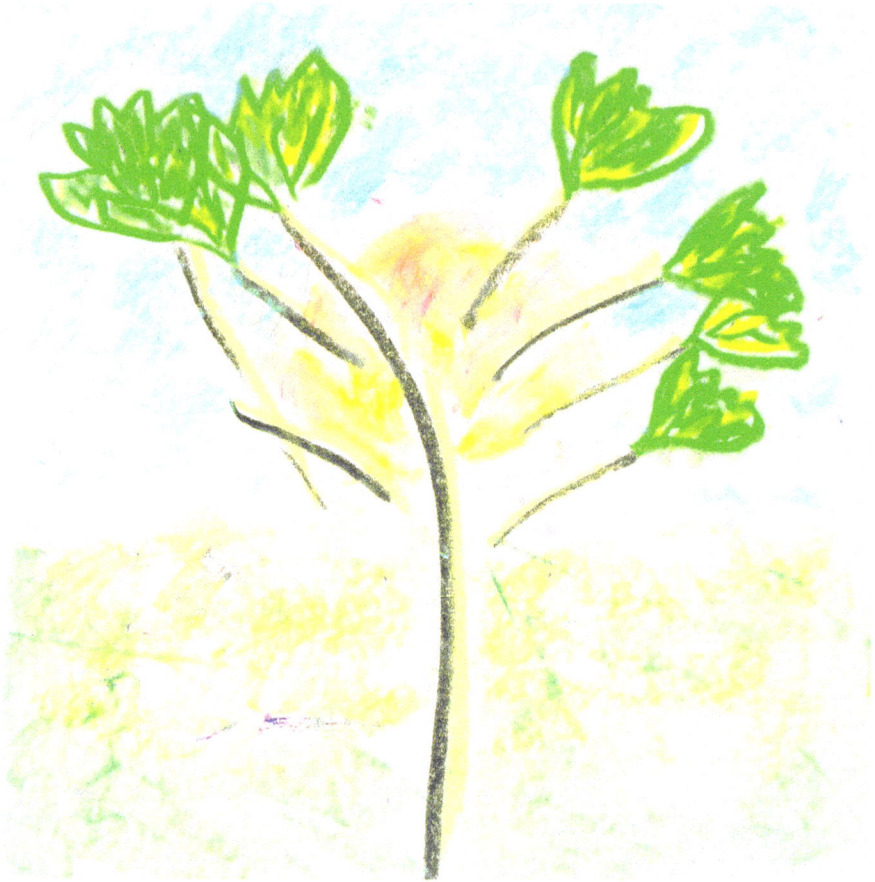

*In the silence between poses,*

*the birds are singing,*

*the refrigerator hums,*

*my wife is dressing for work.*

*A symphony of peace.*

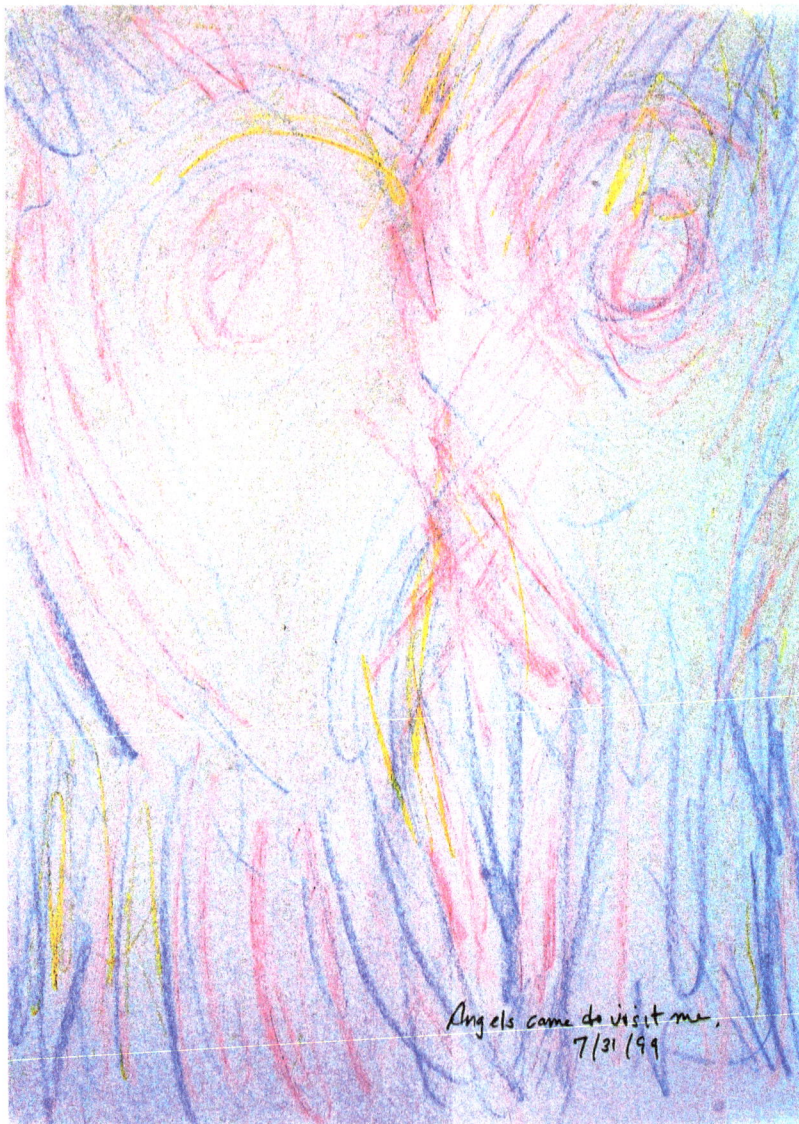

Angels came to visit me,
7/31/99

*I am grateful for all I have been given:*

*The opportunity to see clearly, to hear succinctly,*

*To feel the rhythm of the rain, the joy of plants*

*as first, fat raindrops leave big, wet footprints. (A summer storm)*

*Plants drink deeply, blooming more beautifully when the sun returns.*

*The air is clean and quiet.*

*This is how life flows, giving and receiving, freely and fully,*

*{{{Inside Energy}}} and {{{Inside Love}}}*

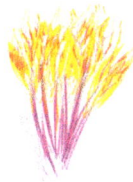

# Fourth Wave

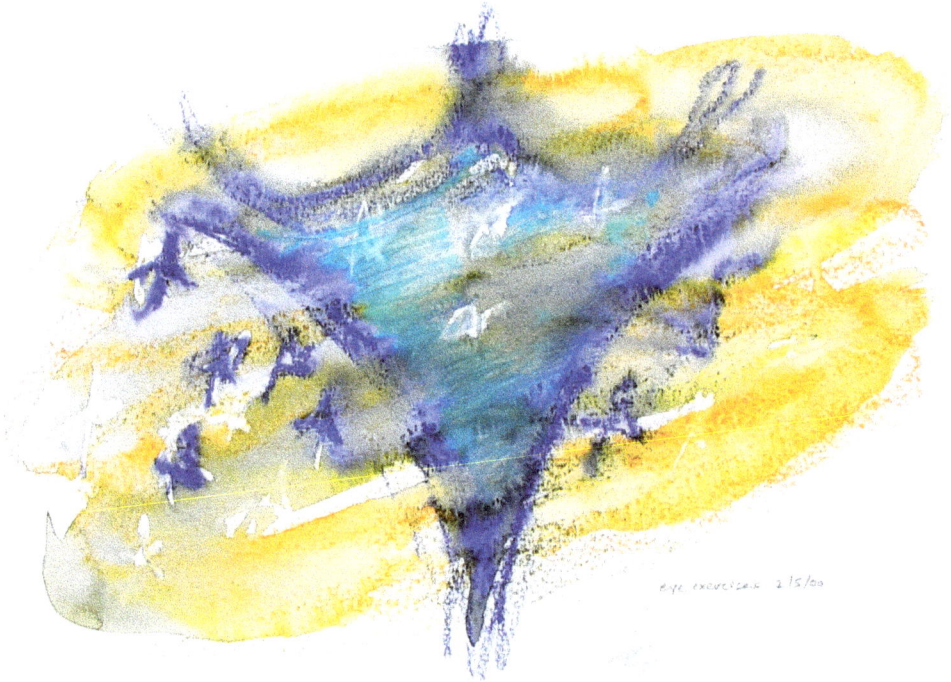

eye exercise 2/5/00

*If the true richness of any moment*

*could be sensed and perceived,*

*all fear and regret*

*would cease to be.*

*In Natarajasana, I am Shiva,*

*the cosmic dancer who*

*creates and destroys the universe*

*in every instant.*

*If the choices I make do not bend*

*toward happiness, then I must bend*

*toward other choices.*

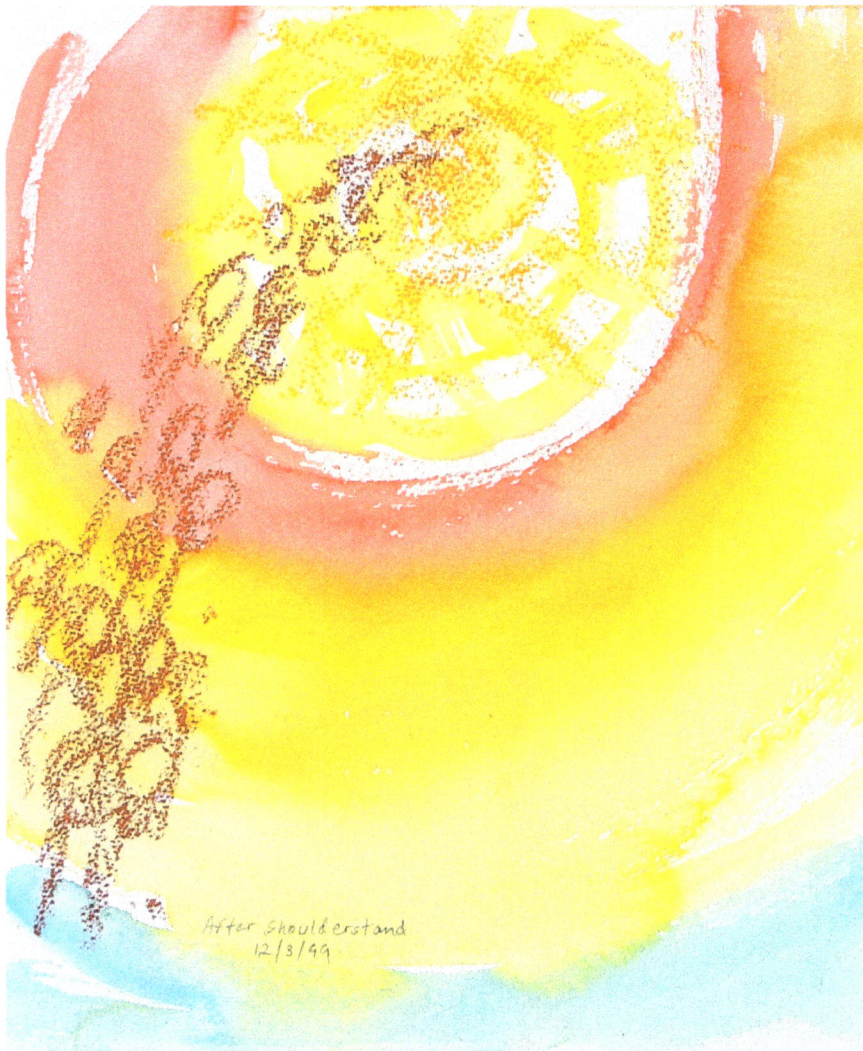

After Shoulderstand
12/3/99

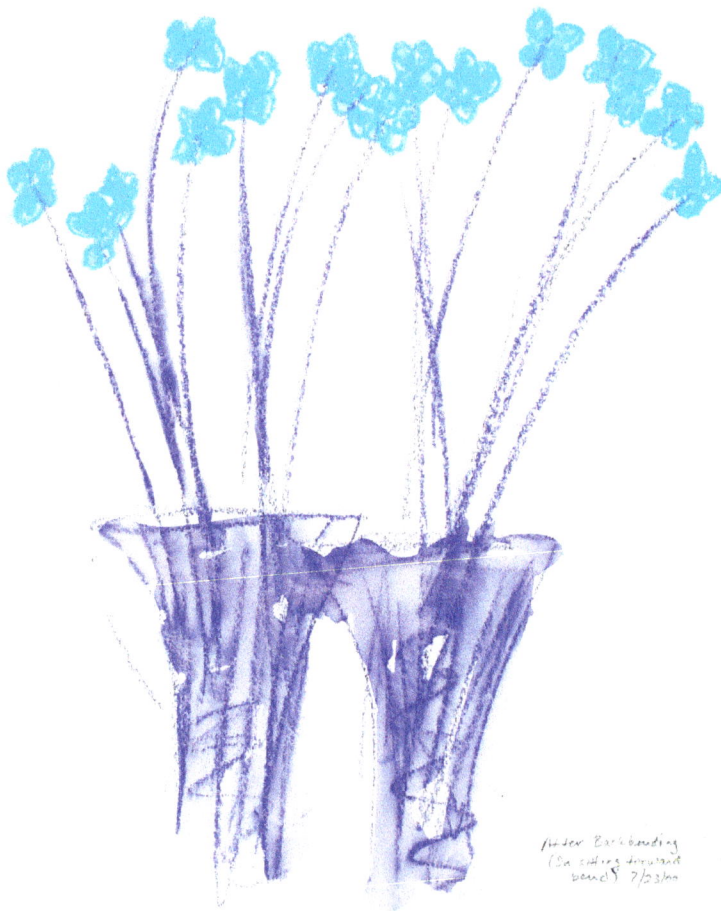

*Death tells me —*

*Move gracefully through your day!*

*Have no fear.*

*All things will be done.*

*When I hurry to finish, little gets done.*

*When I take time to listen, everything is accomplished.*

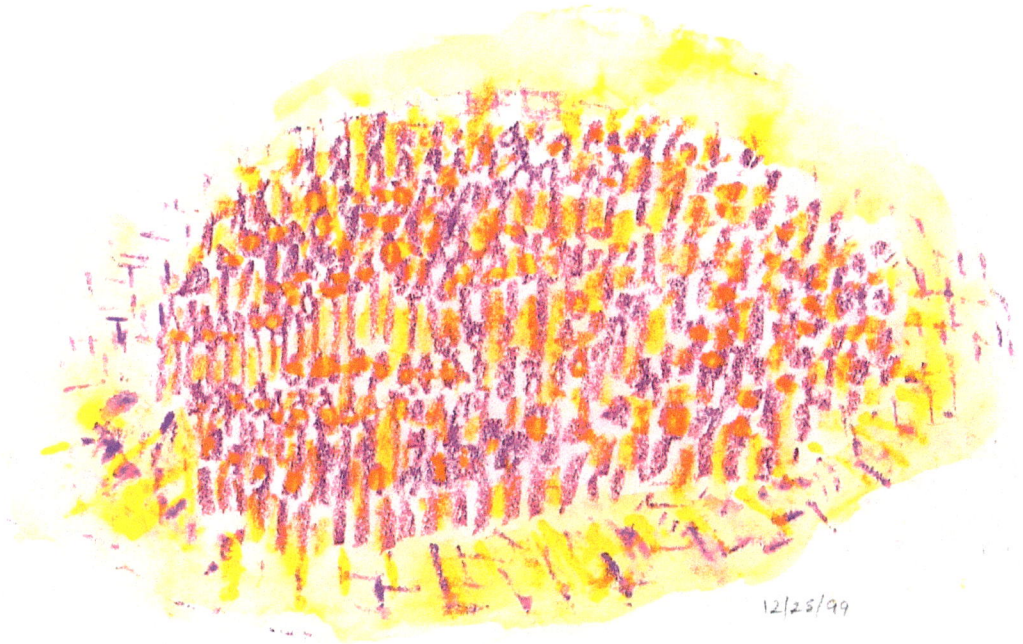

12/28/99

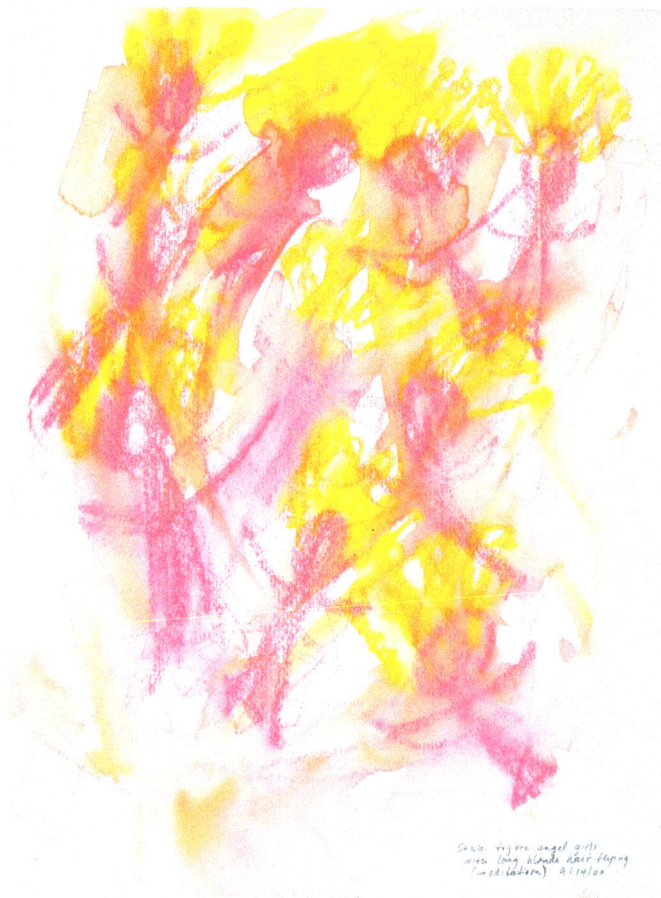

Since rejove angel girls
with long blonde hair flying
(meditation)  9/14/00

*Living richly requires living in the heart of the moment.*

*Here and now, hear, taste, see, smell,*

*sense the infinite variety.*

*Color, sound, form and texture,*

*Richness rings, the echo of the Infinite,*

*from which it all springs.*

*I am laughing inside,*

*resting after Spinal Twist.*


*Laughing*

*because the sprouts and seedlings of life*

*are awakening inside of me.*


*Tickle.*

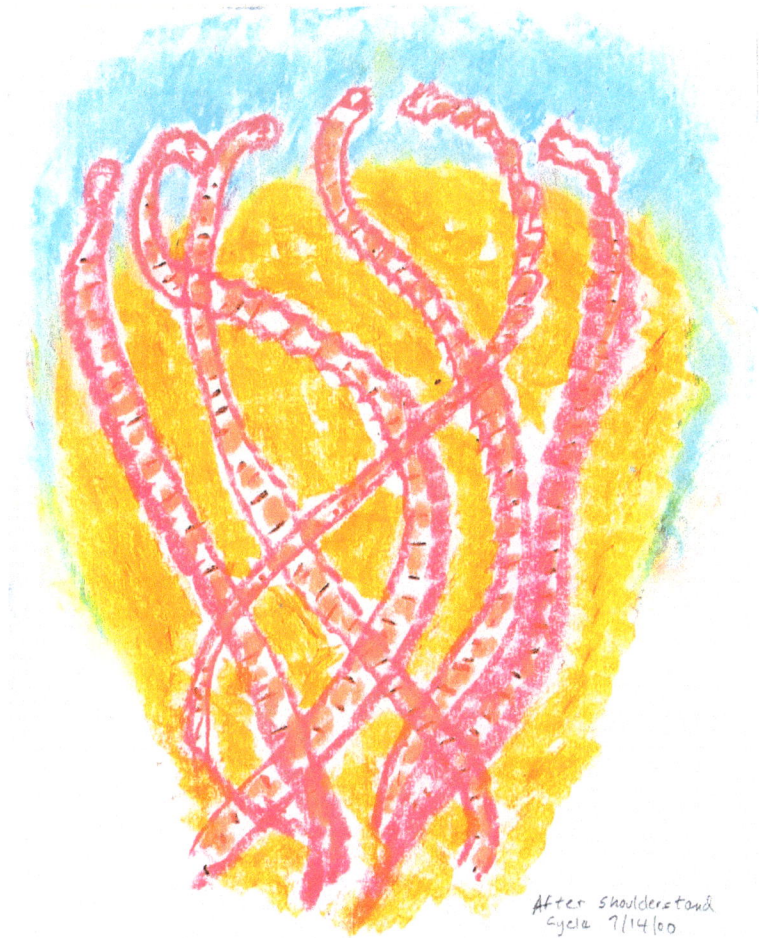

After shoulderstand
cycle 7/14/00

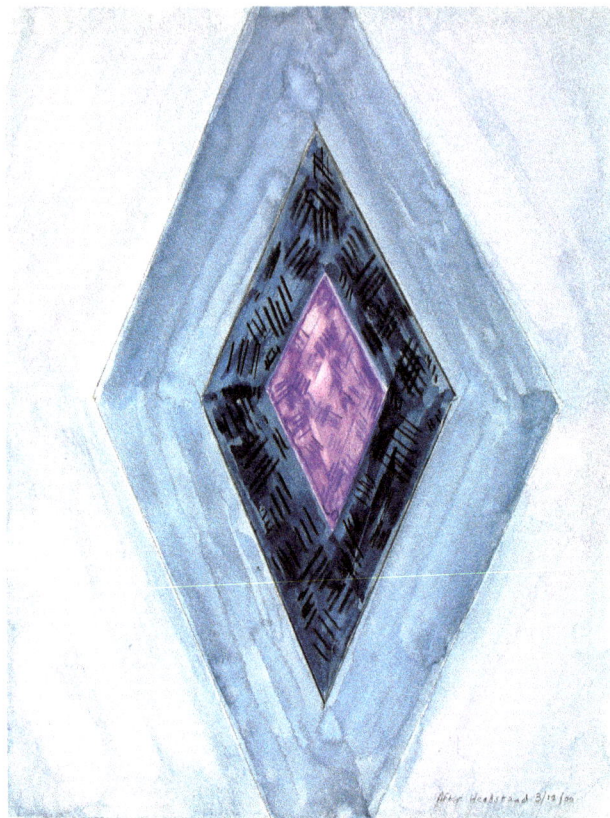

*Inside Yoga*

*After Twisting, my breathing feels beautiful.*

*My back and chest are a diamond kite,*

*tuned and ready to fly.*

FOURTH WAVE

*Experiencing the Infinite lets me flow with the Tao.*

*Flowing with the Tao lets me be with the Infinite.*

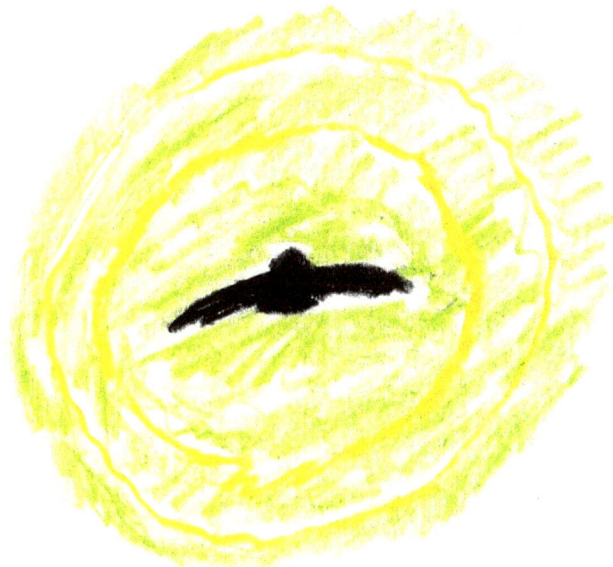

After crow, flying
toward dusk and
quiet darkness.
5/26/99

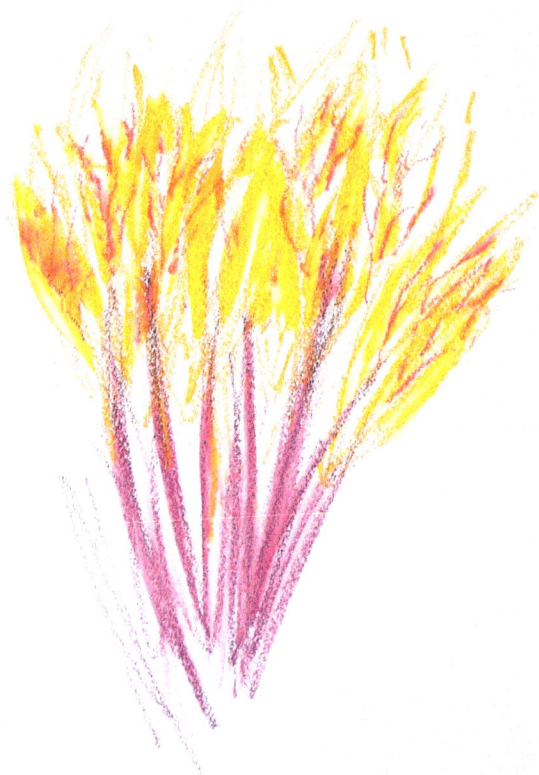

After Shoulderstand cycle
2/23/2000

*Untwisting after Spinal Twist is like gently uncorking a fine wine on a special occasion. As I roll on my back, the richness comes pouring out, perhaps more like mead now, pouring through my heart. It is the nectar in the goblet I once painted, yellow-gold, (like the Princess' hair, only clearer), and in it are flecks of sky blue.*

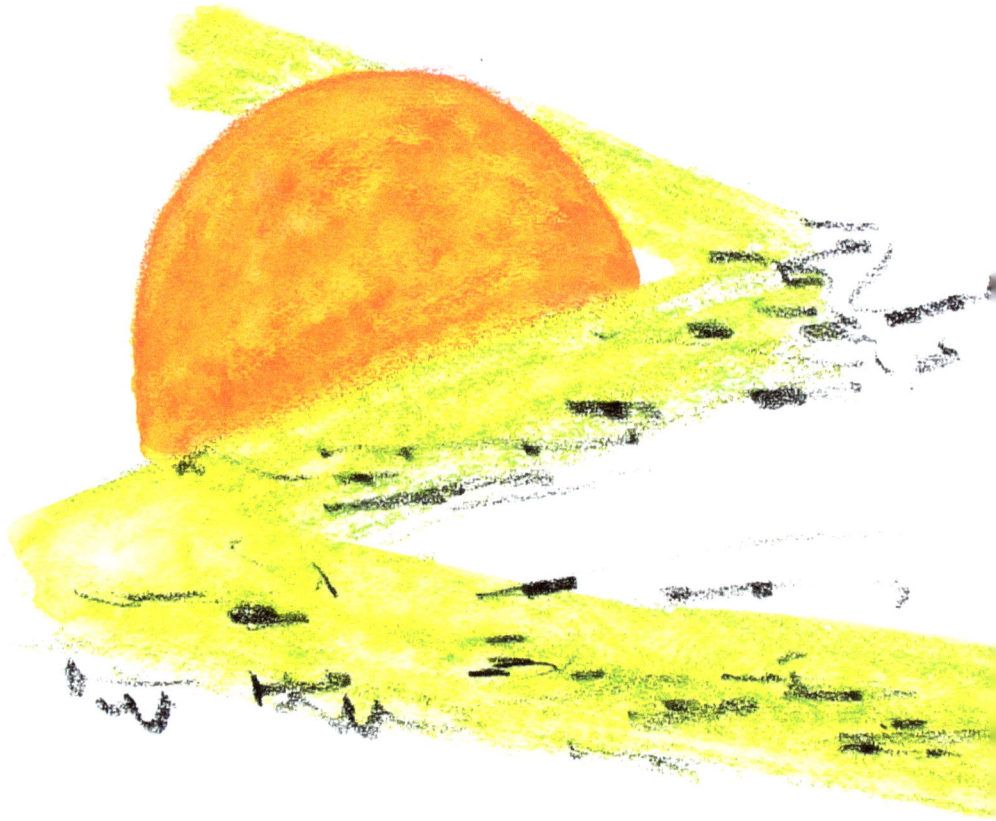

*Today is a good day to die, for I am living!*

*I would prefer to live, but if I die today, I am ready.*

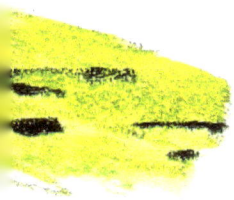

— remembering
9/11/00

*After Fish I see the dragon's fire burning away all crust and crud from the bodies of the Sage. He is smiling, resplendent in red and gold robes and headdress.*

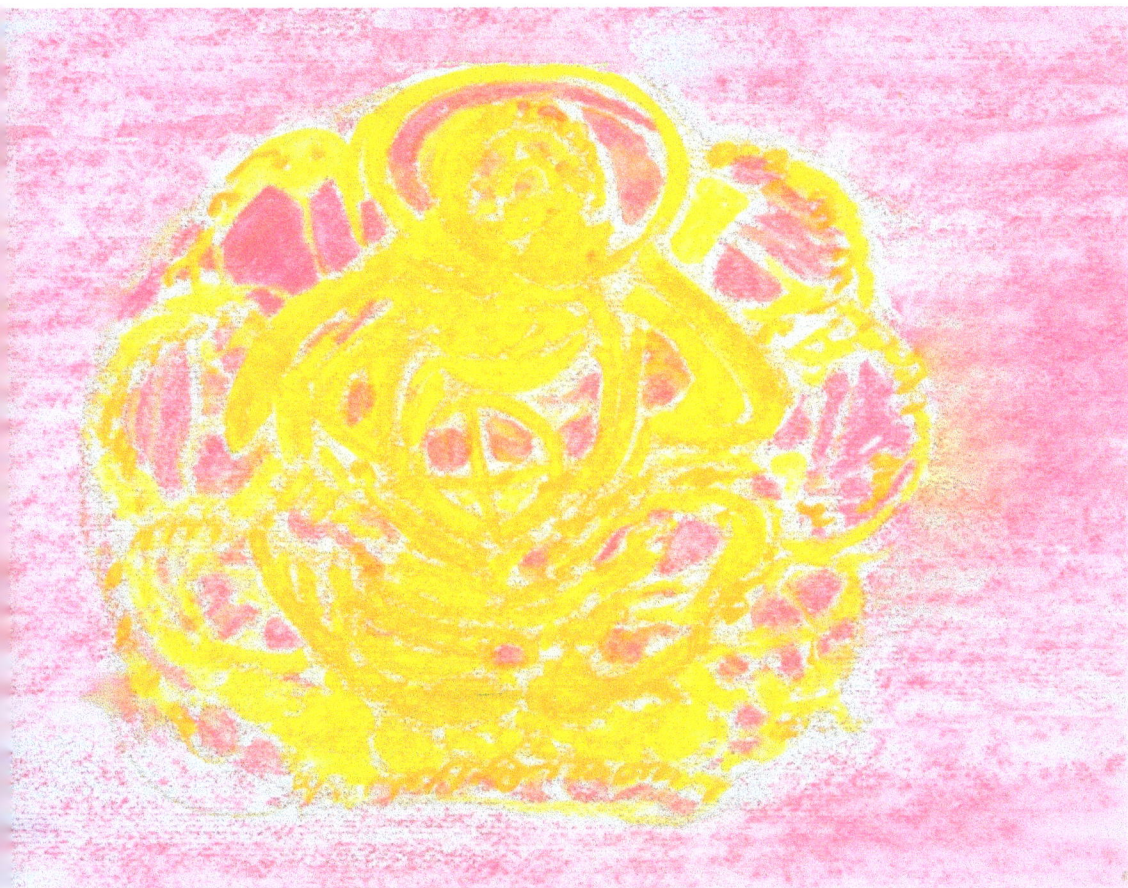

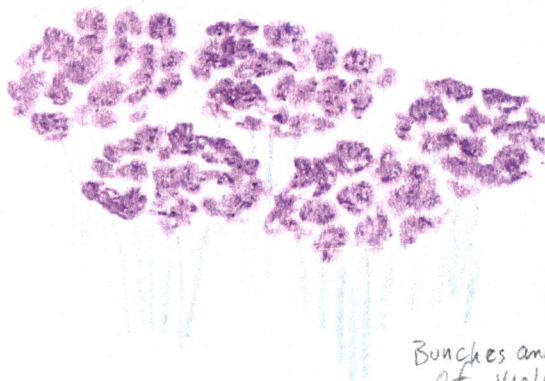

Bunches and Bunches
of Violets.
(After headstand, in
child's pose)
7/15/99

*Youth is even more beautiful now that I am old.*

*(I refer to the growing younger that is now.)*

*…and when I fill my lungs in Alternate Nostril Breathing, and hold, it is not really holding the breath, but floating on top of it, feeling buoyed up by it like a big-chested character balloon in a parade down Main Street.*

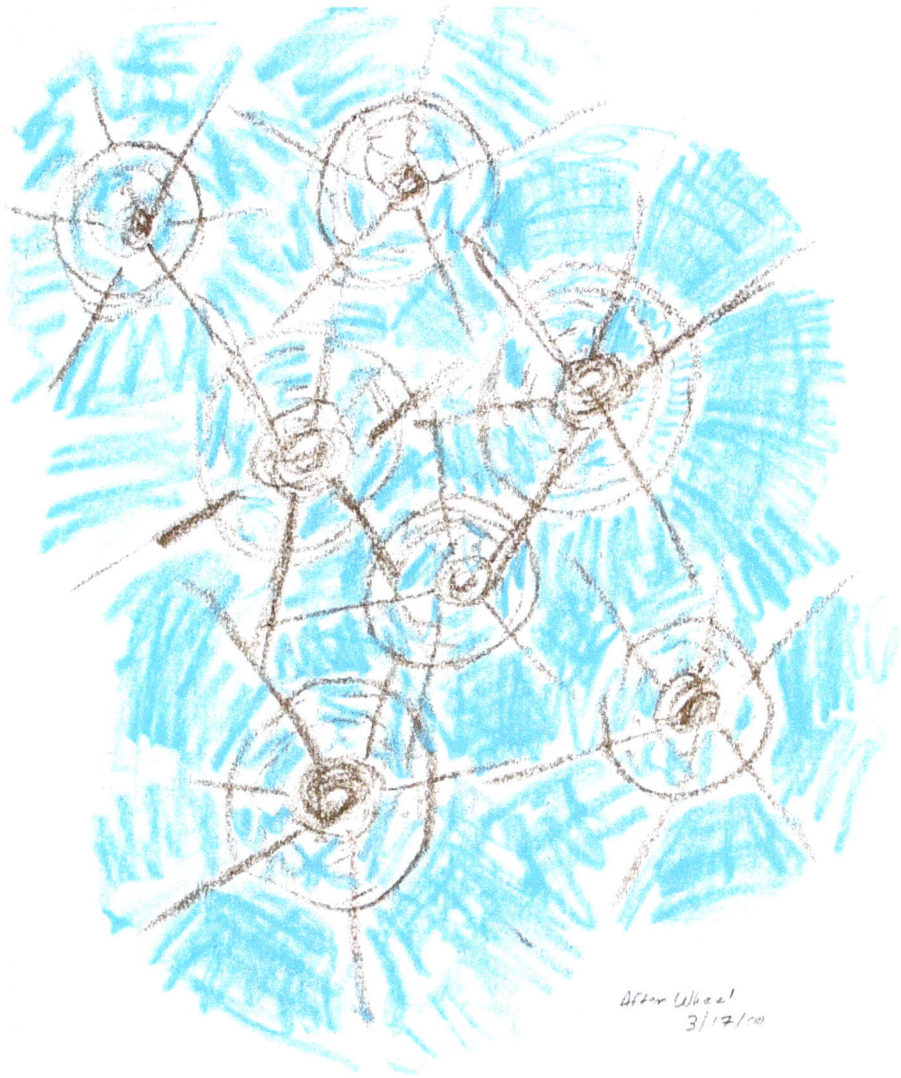

After Wheel
3/17/00

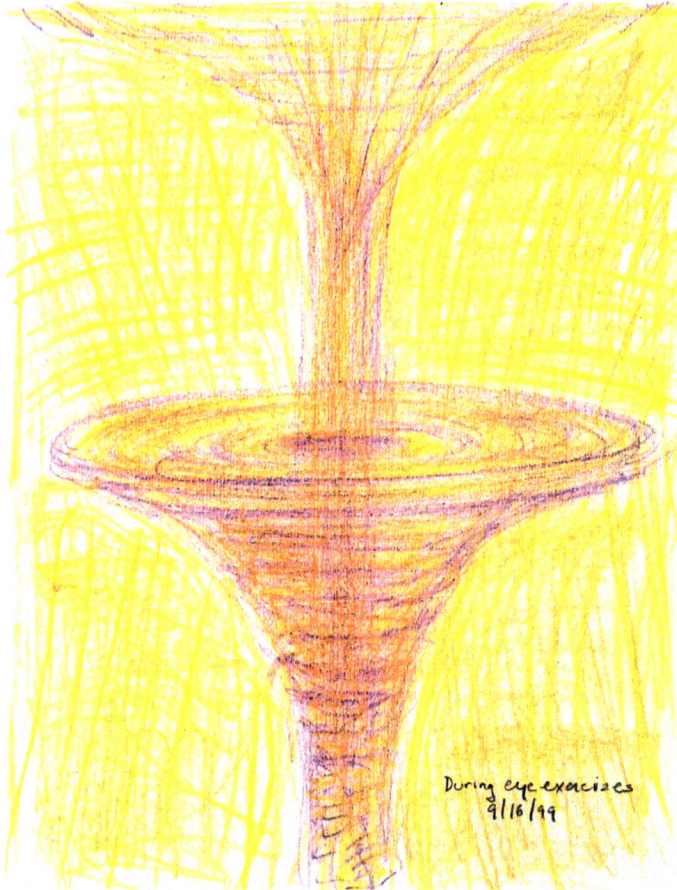

During eye exercises
9/16/99

*Breath informs the body wherein lies its true center,*

*makes obvious the connection to earth and sky.*


*Deeply tethered, grounded in the earth, yet*

*Suspended, buoyed, wafting upwards into the clouds,*

*filling with light and sparkling energy.*

*What is fulfillment for me?*

*If I have to choose,*

*I prefer empty to full.*

*Life is an ever-changing richness of possibilities.*

*I begin each day as an empty glass, waiting*

*to be filled with freshness and newness.*

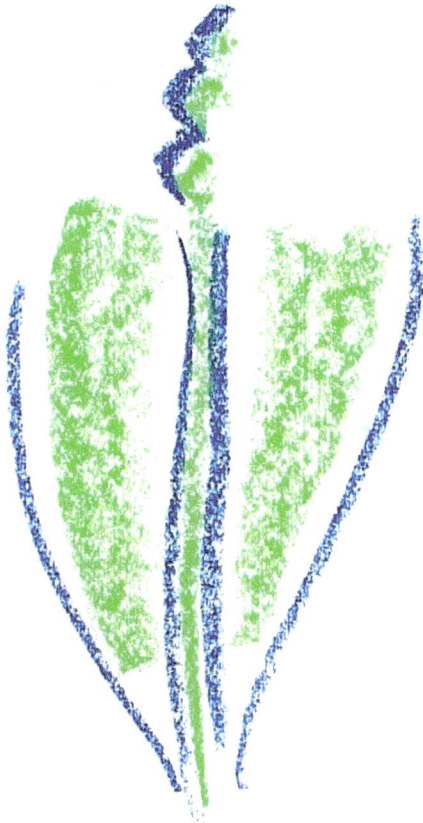

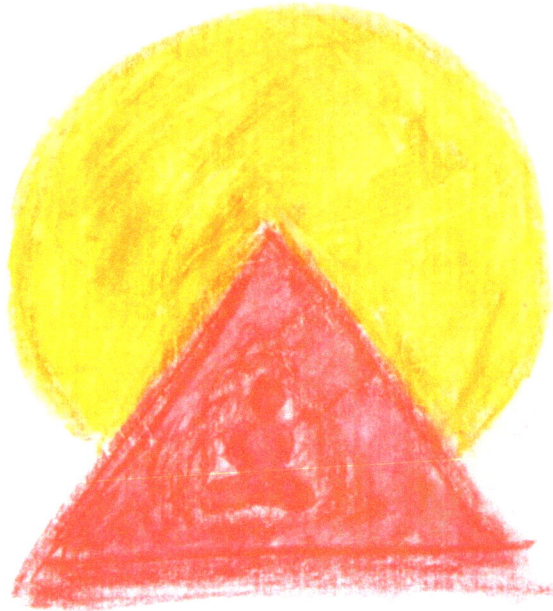

eye exercises (opening)
12/21/00

# Inside Yoga

The world that was dim and distant is near and bright,

full of color; the smoke rises like liquid silk, my back

opening and lengthening with each breath.


"Must have," "must do," "must be doing," disappear.


Here I am in a room at the center of the universe,

my head falling forward and back.

How could I have missed the sparkling sunlight on the leaves?

The gentle sound of the breeze, the delicate notes of the chimes?


Sitting, rooted, listening, breathing.

*A silvertine quiet inside, mirrors*

*the gray and rainy day outside.*


*My body sits itself, shoulders dropping,*

*neck lifting, vertebrae opening, breathing.*


*A simple cross, stuck in the ground*

*absolutely straight, beneath the sky.*


*Breath fills itself, emptying slowly.*

*Sitting, quietly, effortlessly.*

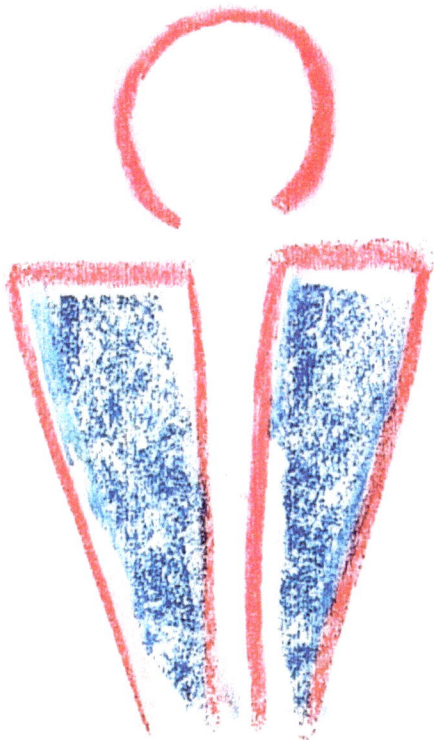

WATCHING THE ENERGY
AFTER HALF SALUTES
(IN MOUNTAIN) 8/11/00

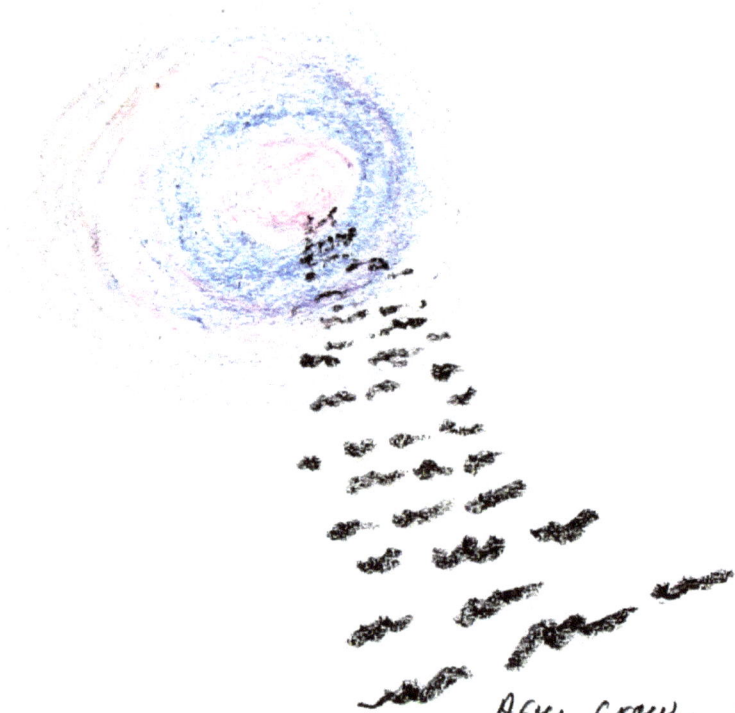

After Crow.
7/31/99

Birds flying
peacefully
toward the
sunset.

*Crow speaks to me*

*of sunsets,*

*and cool, clear*

*open skies,*

*deep, large skies*

*and far, far distances*

*breathing.*

*There is a universe to sail!*

*i am small and light.*

*i float, i fly,*

*i disappear; merging,*

*expanding,*

*being still.*

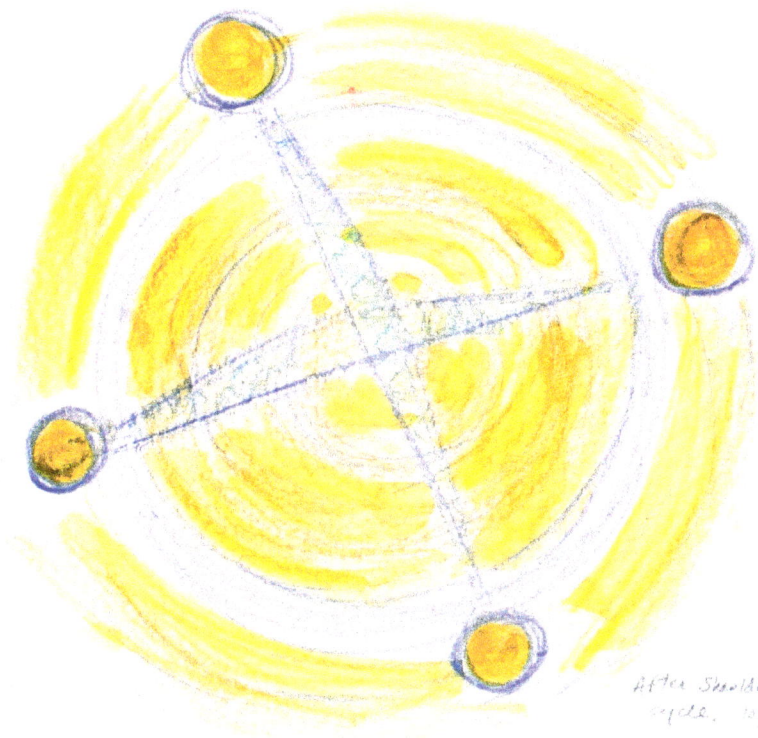

After Shashkasana B
cycle. 10/30/99

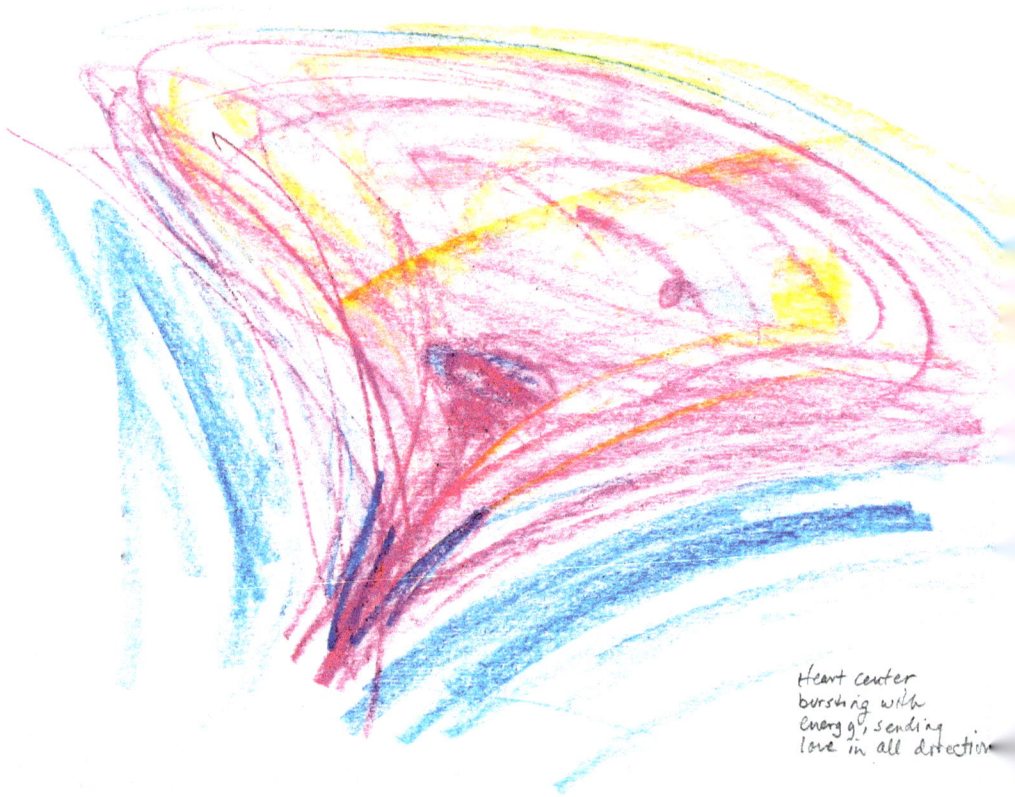

Heart center
bursting with
energy, sending
love in all direction

*i am being shown that my body is like a strong standing stone, and*

*in the center: a densely glowing heart capable of great heat and  power.*


*i am to breathe into this heart, haling it warmer and warmer,*

*letting the love flow out to everyone.*


*the soul is expansive, the heart concentrated, the soul, perhaps (for my*

*purpose), infinitely expansive and moving, like silk in a breeze, around,*

*and in all directions.*

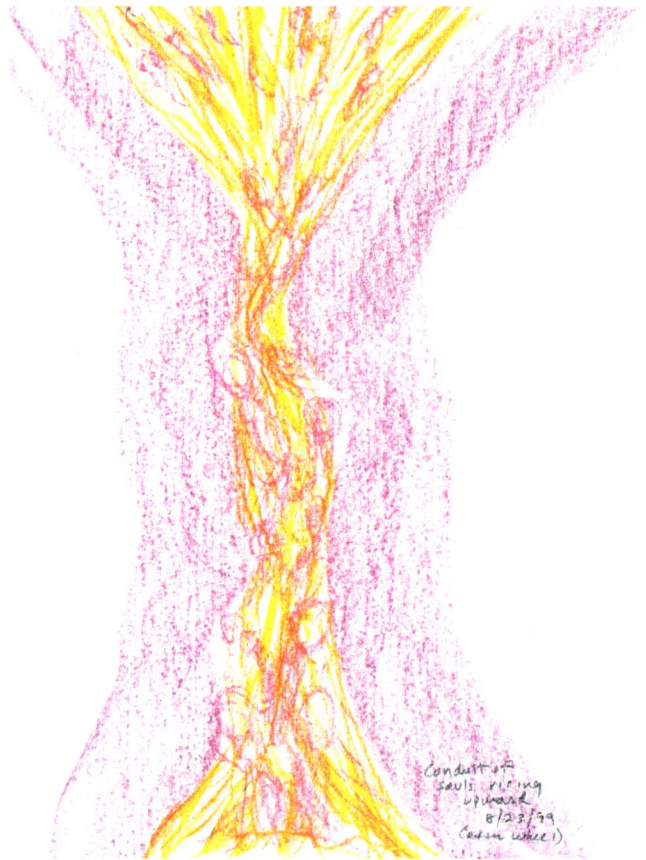

Conduit of
souls rising
upward
8/23/99
(earth wheel)

*I am a conduit and a fountain. My body peels back and away like a flower opening. Where the stamen and pistil would be is my energy-body, shining and shimmering, pulsing and glowing. It is nothing like the body I am used to; does not have the shape of my body, is almost alien in form. (I had no idea it would be like this.)*

*Focusing on my heart center, on the love there, I begin sending love to Charles and to Mary Grace. I notice there is very little difference, or distance between these two entities. They are expansive and nearly touching, like clouds moving gently close to one another. I send love to both and to all.*

*I am aware of my breath and the elastic bands of energy that support me, sitting and breathing. One breath sits suspended at its apex and my eyes roll into the back of my head; I am peaceful. (My head and I are peaceful). I see my body as ashes in a shallow bowl and am aware once again of my energy being, wondering if matter is energy temporarily slowed down. I am thinking that energy cannot be destroyed, so maybe death is an illusion. I am not worried about dying.*

*I am a simple bowl that floats in water.*

*No matter how the wind blows or waves push this way and that,*

*I always come back to my center, a lamp in the night,*

*my refuge, a place of peace.*


*I am a lamp in the night, and my heart*

*its flame.*

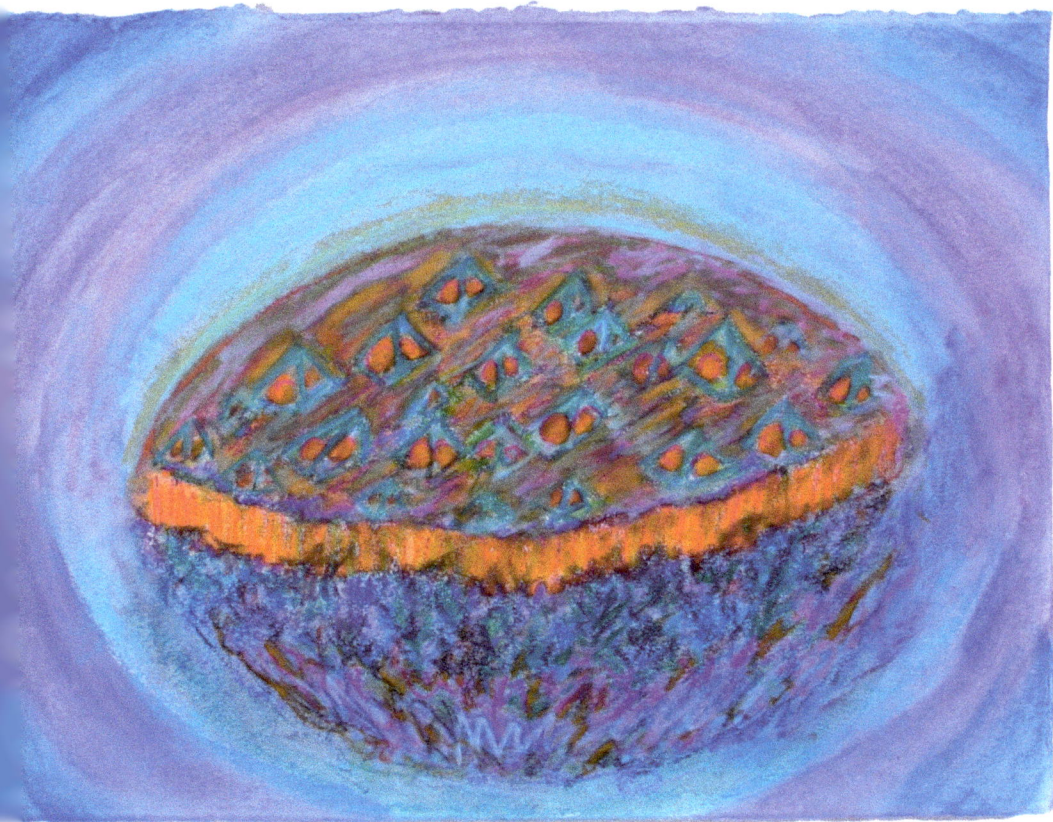

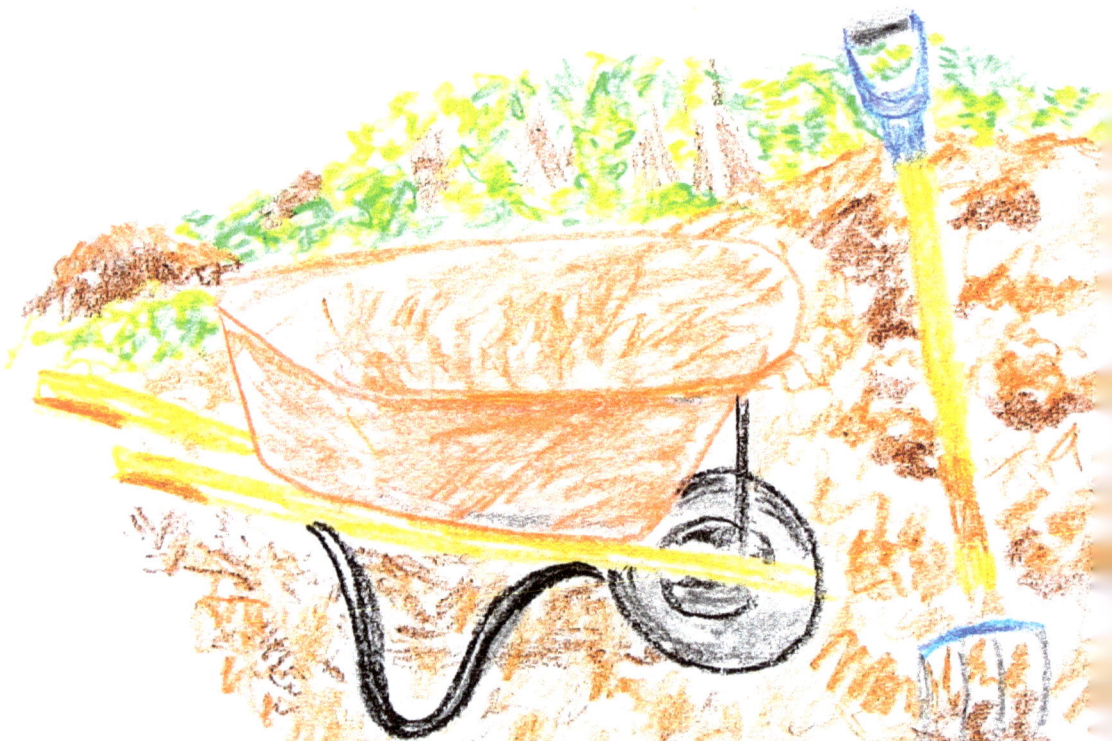

our little orange wheelbarro and
mulchfork outside the window 8/5/99

*I n s i d e   Y o g a*

*The breeze blows, leaves are falling,*

*Insects dart past the window and all is aflutter*

*with the breath and light of the world.*

*Even the mulch-pile sings in warm low tones.*

*Since I woke up, my eyes are open, and my heart feels free,*

*The pyramid of energy has glowed all around me.*

*I have breathed deeply and danced with Shiva,*

*Now it is time to cut the lawn and clean the house.*

*Life so far*

"This is the story of my life so far…" This is the first line of a song by Billy Jonas, a wonderful musician and songwriter in which he gives the highlights, the big stuff, the early inclinations, major turns, people who helped, right up until now, at this moment. So… this is my life so far.

My childhood was comfortable and largely uneventful. I had some musical interest and had a double bass in my hands beginning in the 4th grade, playing in the school orchestra in Roslyn, Long Island, but never having any formal instruction until much later.

By the age of twenty, I was sitting in a damp tent, somewhere in north-central Florida, having dropped out of college, squatting on some other people's communal land with no money, no work, and eating almost all raw food. One morning they woke me up and suggested that I saw some wood to help earn my keep. I was groggy and had little experience with power tools and promptly shoved my left middle finger into the blade of the table saw. In that moment I had no idea how much damage was done, and I heard a voice speak to me, inside my head, clearly saying, "You idiot, you will never play the bass again." That was very interesting, since I had never really taken the instrument seriously or practiced a day in my life.

Suddenly everyone was gone and I stumbled out into a common clearing looking for help. There was a wonderful man there named Golden Sprout and he helped me chew some wheatgrass and comfrey, wrapped it around my injured finger and left me by myself. Immediately I walked across the clearing to the only telephone and called my father, whom I had misused and abused as any post adolescent-adolescent has a tendency to do. I told him that I wanted to go back to school to study the double bass. He said "I don't care what you do as long as you put one foot in front of the other and walk in a direction. It may not lead exactly where you expect, but it will lead somewhere. Come home and we'll make it happen." That was the best advice I have ever had.

Most of my life since then has revolved around studying, performing and teaching the double bass. I completed my Bachelor's and Master's degrees at the University of Miami, studying with the great bassist and pedagogue Dr. Lucas Drew. After college, I spent 21 years in The Florida Orchestra. During the first few years there I married my wife Mary Grace, and she has been my great love and support for all the years since then.

About ten years into my tenure in the orchestra, my back began to hurt and I went to a chiropractor. After his diagnosis and first treatment, I asked him how long I would be coming in for treatments. He said, "For the rest of your life." I said, yeah, no way, and went out and bought a book about Yoga. I took to it right away and I never had any more serious back issues, but what was more fantastic was the new feeling of awareness I was experiencing. I began to write down these impressions as they were happening. During poses and resting between poses wonderful images and phrases were popping into my head and I couldn't ignore them, so I kept a pad and paper with me all the time while I was practicing. At the end of the first year there were 700 pieces of writing, and by the end of the second year, 400 drawings. This book is a selected record of those first moments of awakening.

At around the same time I was introduced to another great double bass teacher named Francois Rabbath, and for the first time I witnessed and heard someone play my instrument the way I might have dreamed it could be played. I felt that I must learn this new way of playing, but it is often difficult, as it is said, "for an old dog to learn new tricks". This is where my yoga practice helped me enormously. I would never touch the bass in the morning, until I had done my yoga practice first. In this way, my mind and body were always clear and open to learning the new technique and I had the patience and discipline to stay with the exercises until my body had learned them. I am convinced that without the relaxed openness that yoga afforded me during this period, I would never have been able to re-learn the double bass in this new way.

After about five years, by the time I began to be able to play simple beautiful melodies on my instrument, I began to hear the same message over and over inside my mind, during my meditations at the end of yoga practice. I felt a strong desire to find some way to do some community service or volunteer work with my instrument.

I went to The Moffitt Cancer Center to offer to play music for patients and was surprised to find that they had established an Arts In Medicine Program and I was invited to come to try playing music for patients in some of the lobbies and waiting rooms. If I wanted to play for individual patients, I would have to take some classes and become a Certified Music Practitioner, and that is what I did. I also entered yoga teacher training and became a Certified Yoga Instructor. I volunteered at Moffitt until I finished my training and was hired by The Arts In Medicine Program where I have been a paid staff member for about 3 years. I occasionally teach gentle yoga classes at the hospital too.

It is quite challenging walking up to someone in the hospital and offering the gift of music in the doorway to their room. It is very different than performing, because it is never supposed to be about me, but about the patient. I must listen carefully to know what music to play and how soft or loud, when to play and when to be quiet and listen; to serve the patient's needs in any way possible both as a healing musician and a sensitive human being. The only way that I maintain my ability to be "in the moment," present and listening for all these important cues, is to keep up my daily yoga practice. The daily yoga practice helps me to renew and refresh myself, remember to breathe, to listen and be grateful for the opportunities that arise in each day of this precious life. I am incredibly grateful for the gift of practice.

I hope you enjoy this book and that in some way it inspires you to rekindle the fire of newness, richness, hope and even joy in your life. As Thich Nhat Hanh says, "It is not a matter of faith, it is a matter of practice." If you do enjoy it, please pass it on, tell your friends and family about Inside Yoga, post it on the web, and help me get this good stuff out there. Thanks.


Lloyd Goldstein
June 1, 2010
www.lloydgoldstein.com

www.ingramcontent.com/pod-product-compliance
Lightning Source LLC
Chambersburg PA
CBHW051559030426
42334CB00031B/3257